Healthy Happy Aging

Yvonne Wagorn
Sonia Théberge
Dr. William A.R. Orban

GSPH

D1501497

Published by

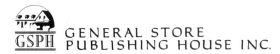
GENERAL STORE
PUBLISHING HOUSE INC.

1 Main Street, Burnstown, Ontario, Canada K0J 1G0
Telephone (613)432-7697   Fax (613)432-7184

ISBN 0-919431-43-7

Printed and bound in Canada.

Designed by Marlene McRoberts and Hugh Malcolm
Illustrated by Hugh Malcolm

General Store Publishing House Inc. gratefully acknowledges the assistance of the Ontario Arts Council.

Canadian Cataloguing in Publication Data

Orban, William A.R.

Healthy happy aging: a positive approach to active living

Issued also in French under title:
Vieillir heureux et en santé: une approche positive à une vie des plus actives

Includes bibliographical references and index.
ISBN 0-919431-43-7

  1.Aged—Health and hygiene. 2. Physical fitness for the aged. 3. Exercise for the aged. 4. Physical education for the aged. 5. Aging. I. Wagorn, Yvonne II. Théberge, Sonia III. Title.

HQ1061.072 1991   613'.0438   C91-090113-9

First Printing April 1991

This book is dedicated to all the seniors involved in the programme Positive Health for Seniors who believed that we were teaching them about aging when, in fact, they were teaching us.

This book was made possible through the financial support of the Seniors Independence Programme, Health & Welfare, Canada, project #4687-5-88/032 and the Élisabeth Bruyère Health Centre, Ottawa.

This book was produced by:

Positive Health for Seniors
Élisabeth Bruyère Health Centre
43 Bruyère Street
Ottawa, Ontario
K1N 5C8
(613) 560-0050

ACKNOWLEDGEMENTS

This book has been a collaborative effort between many people, from well-known specialists in their field to senior citizens in rural Ontario. All were dedicated to this project and each brought a unique and valuable dimension to *Healthy, Happy Aging*. We believe that no other book has had input from so many varied professionals and lay people all with an intense interest in aging and healthy living. Preparation of this final manuscript has taken two years and was produced by a volunteer committee, without whom it would have been impossible.

First, there was our guide and chairperson of this committee **Dr. William A.R. Orban**, retired Professor of Kinanthropology, whose guidance, warmth, dedication and superlative knowledge kept us on track and helped us enjoy every minute of this undertaking. His introduction **What is Aging?** explains his positive attitude to aging and exercise.

Special thanks to several researchers and authors of various chapters in this book who also served as committee members:

Doug Scullion, Teacher's Assistant and Research Assistant in Biomechanics, for research into the aging of body systems, his contribution to the chapter on exercise, and his review of and comments on all that is contained in this manual.

François Gravelle, lecturer in Physical Education and Leisure Studies, University of Ottawa, and,

Dr. J.C. Pageot, Chairman, Department of Leisure Studies, University of Ottawa, for their chapter written specifically for the instructor.

Gilles Hébert, Teacher's Assistant in Psychology, Research Assistant in the field of Sleep and Dreams, for his research and written sections on **Psychological Changes and Attitudes** and **Quality of Life**.

Thanks to the students employed during the summer of 1990:

Christine Dalgity, St. Lawrence College; **Paul Wagorn**, University of Waterloo; **Pamela Willis**, University of Victoria, for research and preparation of **Living with Aging, Section 1**, **Common Disorders**, and the **Glossary** and for their patience and good humour during a hectic summer.

A very special thanks to **Dianne Parker-Taillon**, Director of Physiotherapy, Ottawa General Hospital, whose conscientious review of and invaluable input to this complete manual, especially the exercise chapter, has ensured the quality which we strived so hard to maintain.

Many thanks to the rest of the members of our team; we couldn't have achieved these results without you:

Rolland Champagne, fitness instructor, Positive Health for Seniors, Wendover, Ontario,

Dale Edwards, Coordinator, Back Care Programme, Élisabeth Bruyère Health Centre,

Henri Groulx, participant, Positive Health for Seniors, Hawkesbury, Ontario,

Sharon Hudson, Coordinator, Senior Programmes, YM/YWCA,

Jean Hurtubise, participant, Positive Health for Seniors, Vankleek Hill, Ontario,

Thérèse Larocque, fitness instructor, Positive Health for Seniors, Hawkesbury, Ontario, and

Aubert Séguin, participant, Positive Health for Seniors, Vankleek Hill, Ontario.

To **Janet Chambers,** Manager, Senior Services, Canadian Red Cross Society, **Jennifer Godfrey**, Fun 'n Fitness Officer, Canadian Red Cross Society and **Norma Strachan**, Project Manager, Medication Awareness Project, Council on Aging, Ottawa-Carleton, thank you for your input.

Hats off to **Christine Gardner** who was always able to take our written notes, make sense of them and produce a legible manuscript.

Grateful appreciation to the staff at Élisabeth Bruyère Health Centre, especially **Donna Lordon**, Assistant Executive Director of Clinical Services, who stood behind this project from the beginning to the end.

Thanks to our publishing team from **General Store Publishing House**, **Tim Gordon**, Publisher, **Marlene McRoberts**, Designer and **Hugh Malcolm**, Illustrator, for their expertise, guidance and patience.

Without funding from **Seniors Independence Programme**, **Health & Welfare, Canada**, and the guidance provided by **Rita Lemick**, Programme Officer, Health Promotion Directorate, Health and Welfare, Canada, this book would not be available to you so that you may experience *Healthy, Happy Aging*.

Sincere appreciation to the organizations and individuals who reviewed the manuscript:

The Arthritis Society and,

Dr. C. Doug Smith, Rheumatologist, Ottawa General Hospital (Arthritis),

Dr. Yvan Lavoie, (Diabetes, Problems with the Heart and Circulatory System),

Sylvie Théberge, (Psychological Changes and Attitudes, Quality of Life), and

Pauline Witherly-Manuel, Public Relations, OSTOP Ottawa, Osteoporosis Support Group (Osteoporosis).

Last but not least, to all the seniors involved in the programme Positive Health for Seniors who allowed us to field test this manual with them, and for their support, enthusiasm and involvement in this programme. This manual is for you!

Yvonne Wagorn
Yvonne Wagorn

Sonia Théberge
Sonia Théberge

TABLE OF CONTENTS

CHAPTER 2: COMMON PHYSICAL DISORDERS

CHAPTER 3: LIVING WITH AGING

FOREWORD

This book was produced by the programme Positive Health for Seniors, a bilingual outreach health promotion project that trains seniors to become leaders of their peers in physical activity. This programme has evolved through many years from a simple fitness programme to a programme that includes many components: fitness, education, leadership and social interaction. It was through working closely with the senior population that we came to realize that as we age, we understand very little of what happens to our bodies and what steps we may take to improve our quality of life.

This book offers you, the reader, the opportunity to understand aging and to develop strategies to make sure that you actually *enjoy* the aging process.

The topics presented in this book are for all age groups. We are all aging; some have just been aging longer than others.

Included in the exercise chapter are fitness programmes that will benefit those who have never been introduced to exercise and those who have managed to maintain a proper level of fitness. Make these programmes part of your life and enjoy the positive effects that they will bring.

If you work with older adults, we have not forgotten you. You will gain great insight into the aging body and, to complement your new knowledge, we have included a chapter just for you on planning and designing a fitness class for seniors.

While reading this book, you will be introduced to two characters, Alice and Albert. Follow them; they will lead you through the chapters, exercise with you and become your mentors as you proceed. You will not be alone in your quest for healthy living — Alice and Albert will always work out with you.

Read this book with pleasure. It was meant for that purpose. We believe it will start you on the road to *HEALTHY, HAPPY AGING*.

WHAT IS AGING?

Aging is a process of accumulating experiences, enriching our lives through knowledge and physical skills.

This acquired wisdom gives us the potential to make sensible and beneficial decisions about ourselves.

The fullness and richness of our remaining years is in our hands. Barring accidents and disease the quality of our golden years is resolved primarily by ourselves. The more we control our lives the more enjoyable the remaining years can be.

The degree of independence we have in our lives is directly related to how active we are in body, mind and spirit.

In spite of some decreases in efficiency and capacity with increasing age, a relatively high level of physical and mental function can be maintained for years.

We have a choice: a choice to give up our independence and fade away or to take control and remain vigorously active fully enjoying our remaining years.

Use it or lose it is a rule that applies to our bodies and minds. It is even more significant as we age since we gradually lose intellectual and physical capacity with increasing years.

Keeping mentally and physically active reduces the rate at which we lose our functions and enables us to more fully enjoy and increase the quality of the golden years of our life.

The physical fitness programme and information provided in this book is written specifically for you. If you follow it according to the instructions, it will keep you physically active and give you increased zest for living.

CHAPTER 1

HOW YOUR BODY AGES

How your body ages is not exactly clear, however it is known that the process of aging differs from person to person as well as from one body system (heart, lungs, muscles, etc.) to another.

The main factors that influence the aging of your body are time, heredity and your surroundings over which you have very little control. There are, however, other aspects of your life such as diet, lifestyle and level of exercise which can positively benefit the aging process and increase your quality of life and well being.

This chapter takes a look at the natural aging process of your body with emphasis on the benefits as well as the possible hazards that may be encountered with exercise. As much as exercise can be beneficial for maintaining a healthy body, it is very important to listen to the various signs that your body may send you when you are exercising too hard or improperly.

The chapter is broken down into seven sections in order to help you understand the seven different systems that make up your wonderful body, as well as how each of these is affected by aging and exercise.

Section 1

YOUR BRAIN AND NERVES
(THE NERVOUS SYSTEM)

What is the nervous system ?

- the nervous system consists of the brain, the spinal cord and all the *nerves* that travel through the body

What does it do ?
The brain:

- is thought to be the centre of intellect and reasoning, and may also play a major role in controlling thoughts and emotions

The nervous system controls:

- the senses (seeing, hearing, smelling, touching and tasting)

- body movements

- all the *organs* of the body

- coordination

How does this happen ?

- messages travel through the nerves from the brain to different parts of the body and back to the brain to control the senses, *muscles* and organs

- thinking and reasoning are accomplished by messages travelling between different parts of the brain

In the nervous system...

aging causes:

- a decrease in the number of brain and nerve *cells*

- a slowing down of messages travelling along the nerves

- a decrease in *blood flow* to the nervous system

...so you may notice:

- a slower reaction time

- a decrease in balance and coordination

- slower movements

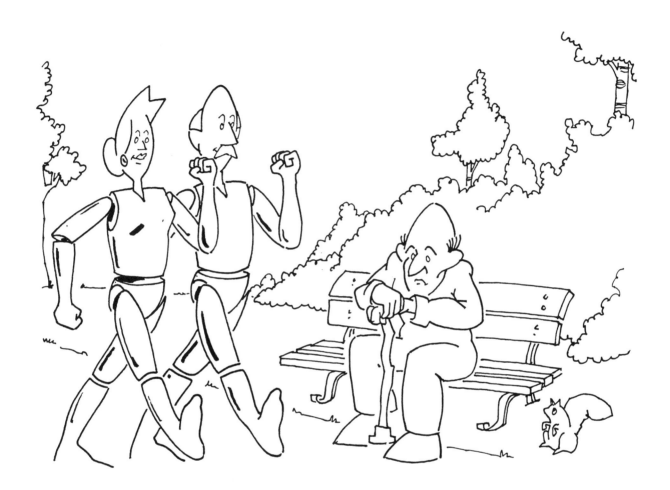

- a decrease in attention and concentration

- an increase in the length of time it takes to understand ideas

- a decrease in emotional control

- a gradual loss of short-term memory

What regular exercise may do for you:

- increase blood flow to the brain

- maintain the flow of messages travelling along the nervous system

- increase self-confidence

In the eyes...

aging causes:

- a thickening and hardening of the *cornea*

- a loss of liquid inside the eyeball

- the *pupil* to become smaller

- a decrease in the number of cells in the eye

- a decrease in blood flow to the eye

- a decrease in the size and strength of muscles that control eye movement

...so you may notice:

- a difficulty in adapting to light and dark

- a difficulty in distinguishing certain colours

- blurred vision

- a difficulty in focusing on objects

- a squinting of the eyes

- a decrease in *peripheral vision* i.e. *field of vision*

- a loss of balance

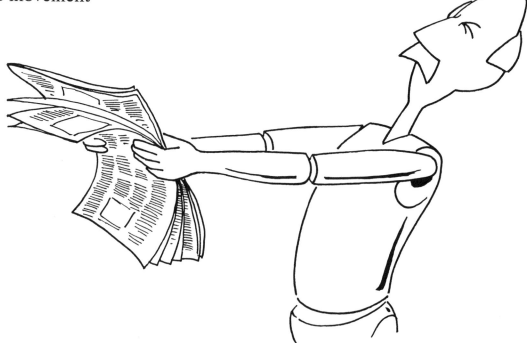

In the ears...

aging causes:
- a decrease in blood flow to the ear
- a narrowing of the *ear canal*
- a decrease in function in the part of the ear that controls balance

...so you may notice:
- a difficulty in hearing
- a difficulty in locating the source of sounds
- a difficulty in understanding someone who speaks quickly
- a difficulty in hearing high-pitched sounds and voices
- a decrease in balance

Things to remember when you exercise:
- practise balance and coordination exercises
- be aware of your arm and leg positions in space when you exercise
- when you exercise in a group, be aware of other people and objects around you
- always exercise in well lit areas
- if you exercise to music, be sure that the mood of the music complements the exercise

DO NOT:
- do not perform quick movements or change direction of movement quickly (this may cause loss of balance or dizziness)

Warning signs of excessive exercise

Stop exercising when:
- you feel an unusual loss of balance
- you sense a "ringing" in your ears
- your ears feel blocked

Section 2

YOUR HEART, BLOOD VESSELS AND BLOOD (THE CARDIOVASCULAR SYSTEM)

What is the cardiovascular system ?

- the cardiovascular system consists of the heart, *blood vessels* and blood

What does it do ?

- it supplies the body with *oxygen* from the lungs

- it supplies the body with *nutrients* from the digestive system (see section 6)

- it transports *carbon dioxide* and other waste products out of the body

How does this happen ?

- the heart muscle contracts, causing blood to flow through the blood vessels

- the blood vessels help the flow of blood by expanding and contracting

- the blood picks up oxygen at the lungs and carries it to the rest of the body where it is used

- nutrients are picked up by the blood from the intestines and carried to the rest of the body

- the blood picks up carbon dioxide and other waste products from the body and carries them away

In the cardiovascular system...

aging causes:

- a decrease in the number of heart muscle cells

- a decrease in the strength of the heart muscle

- a decrease in the *elasticity* of the heart muscle

- a decrease in blood flow to the heart muscle

- the heart valves to become stiffer

- a decrease in the elasticity of the blood vessels

- fatty deposits to appear in the blood vessels (cholesterol)

- calcium deposits to appear in the blood vessels

- an increase in the resistance to blood flow

- a decrease in blood flow to some organs

- an increased vulnerability to minor internal bleeding

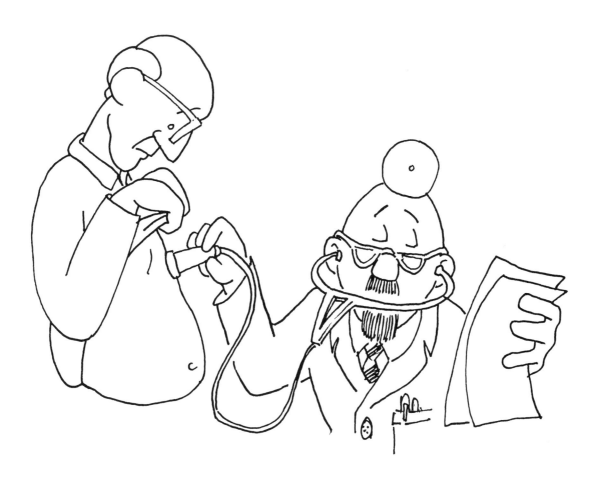

...so you may notice:

- a decrease in *resting heart rate*

- a rapid increase in *heart rate* during physical activity

- an increase in *blood pressure*

- shortness of breath

- *chronic* fatigue

- a loss of balance

- a sense of dizziness

- paleness or redness of the skin

- a decrease in the function of some organs

- *varicose veins*

- a numbing of limbs, fingers and toes

- a coldness of limbs, fingers and toes

- an increase in sensitivity to cold

What regular exercise may do for you:

- increase the strength of heart muscle

- increase blood flow to some organs

- increase *endurance*

- improve overall breathing

- decrease blood pressure

- increase the ability to recover after physical activity

- improve the efficiency of the heart

- increase blood flow to the heart

- decrease heart rate during exercise

- improve overall blood flow

Things to remember when you exercise:

- see your doctor before exercising especially if you have ever experienced cardiovascular problems (*heart attacks, strokes, angina*) or if you are taking any medication

- be aware of your breathing when you exercise (don't forget to breathe!)

- always exercise at your own pace (don't overdo it!)

- watch out for changes in facial colouring (paleness, excessive flushing)

- allow a recovery period between each high intensity exercise

- try to exercise with a partner and perform the *talk test* (if you can't keep up a conversation, you're exercising too hard!)

- make sure that you know when to breathe in and breathe out during an exercise

- take your *resting, exercising* and *recovery pulse rates*, and compare them to your *target heart rate*

- do exercises that gradually increase your heart rate

- do exercises that gradually increase your breathing rate

- always allow for a relaxation period at the end of exercising

DO NOT:

- do not do exercises which involve holding one's breath, i.e. the *Valsalva manoeuvre*

- do not do exercises that restrict movement of the chest

- do not allow your head to drop below your waist when exercising

- do not do *prolonged strength exercises*

- do not change the tempo of your exercising too quickly

- do not exercise in temperatures which are too cold or too hot

- do not do cross-legged exercises

- do not do overhead arm exercises if you are overly fatigued

- never stand or sit still immediately after exercising

Warning signs of excessive exercise

Stop exercising when:

- you feel excessive fatigue
- you find that you cannot talk
- your skin gets excessively pale or red
- you feel a loss of balance
- you experience extreme behavioural changes, i.e. aggresiveness
- you notice that you are sweating excessively
- you start to shiver
- you experience a temporary loss of speech, trouble in speaking or trouble in understanding speech
- you get a nosebleed
- you feel dizzy
- you feel nauseous
- you feel pain in the shoulders, chest, arms, neck or jaw
- you experience a sudden weakness or numbing of the face, arms or legs
- you feel abdominal pain
- you feel irregular heartbeats
- you experience a change in vision
- you experience double vision
- you experience headaches

Section 3

YOUR BONES AND MOVABLE JOINTS
(THE SKELETAL SYSTEM AND JOINTS)

What is the skeletal system ?

- the skeletal system consists of all the bone and *cartilage* in the body

What are the movable joints?

- the movable *joints* consist of a meeting of two bones, cartilage, *ligaments, tendons* and other *tissues*

What does it do ?
The skeletal system:

- supports the body

- protects the brain, *spinal cord* and other organs (lungs, heart) from injury

The movable joints:

- allow for movement of different parts of the body

- attach the bones together

How does this happen ?

- the bones of the body act as a frame which supports the body

- parts of the skeletal system surround and protect most major organs (skull, pelvis, rib cage, *vertebral column*)

- movement is produced by the contraction and relaxation of muscles across a joint

The parts which make up a movable joint are:

- cartilage — allows for bone to bone contact

- ligaments — attach the bones together at a joint

- tendons — attach muscles to bones

In the skeletal system...

aging causes:

- a decrease in the amount of bone tissue

- a decrease in *bone density*

- a decrease in the amount of *calcium* in the bone tissue

- a slow-down in replacement of bone tissue

- possible narrowing of the joint space

- possible fluid changes in the joints

- possible bony growths in the joints

- stiffening of the ligaments

- fraying of the cartilage

- a decrease in the elasticity of cartilage

...so you may notice:

- an increase in vulnerability to bone fractures

- a decrease in height

- a poorer posture

- a decrease in *flexibility*

- a decrease in joint stability

- a deformation of bone tissue at the joint

- a swelling at the joints

- an increase in joint pain (arthritis — see ch. 2)

- an increase in the cracking sound at the joint

- a loss of balance

What regular exercise may do for you:
- increase joint flexibility

- increase joint stability

- increase bone strength

- decrease vulnerability to bone fractures

- improve posture

Things to remember when you exercise:

- do flexibility and full *range of motion* exercises for all joints (small and large)

- always maintain good posture

- keep the room in which you are exercising at a comfortable temperature

- consult your doctor for specific exercises if you have joint or arthritic pain (see ch. 2)

- use mats for floor exercises

- use slow rhythmic movements when exercising

DO NOT:

- do not perform exercises with quick, sharp movements, i.e. *ballistic movements*

- do not perform exercises which produce large shocks to the bones, e.g. jumping jacks

- do not exercise if excessive joint or bone pain persists

- do not exercise if joint swelling occurs

- do not do head rotations behind the shoulder (full head rotations)

- do not perform exercises which place too much weight on the joints, e.g. kneeling exercises

- do not exercise with your knees locked

Warning signs of excessive exercise

Stop exercising when:

- swelling occurs in the joints

- you feel pain in the bones or joints

Section 4

YOUR MUSCLES
(THE MUSCULAR SYSTEM)

What is the muscular system ?
- the muscular system consists of all the muscles in the body

What does it do ?
- it supports the body and is responsible for posture
- it holds the bones together
- it is responsible for all body movements
- it produces body heat
- it helps some organs (bowels, stomach) to function efficiently
- it protects the body from injury

How does this happen ?
- continuous partial contraction of the muscles helps the body stay in an upright position

- body movement is achieved through contraction of the muscles which are attached to the bones by the tendons
- body heat is produced and released throughout the body when muscles contract
- organ function is helped by the contraction of muscles which massage and place a demand on the organ
- muscles act as protection from injury by acting as a cushion between the body and the environment

In the muscular system...
aging causes:
- a decrease in the number of muscle cells
- a decrease in the size of muscle cells

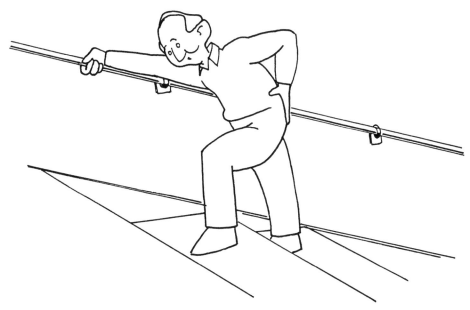

- an increase in the water and fat content of muscle

- a decrease in blood flow to the muscles

- a decrease in the speed of muscle contractions

- a decrease in the ability of muscles to receive messages from the brain

- a decrease in the elasticity of muscles

- the muscles to become injured more easily

- the muscles to become less able to repair themselves

...so you may notice:

- a decrease in muscle size

- a loss of muscle firmness

- a decrease in muscle strength

- a decrease in muscle endurance

- an increase in muscle cramps and soreness

- a decrease in the control and speed of movements

- a loss of balance

- a decrease in flexibility

- an increase in muscle injuries

- an increased difficulty in digestion

- a decrease in bladder control

- a decrease in bowel control

What regular exercise may do for you:

- increase muscle size

- firm up the body

- increase muscle strength

- increase muscle endurance

- improve coordination

- increase flexibility

- increase blood flow to the muscles

- decrease muscle injuries

- improve digestion and excretion

- increase bladder control

Things to remember when you exercise:

- always try to keep good posture

- do stretching exercises for all *muscle groups*

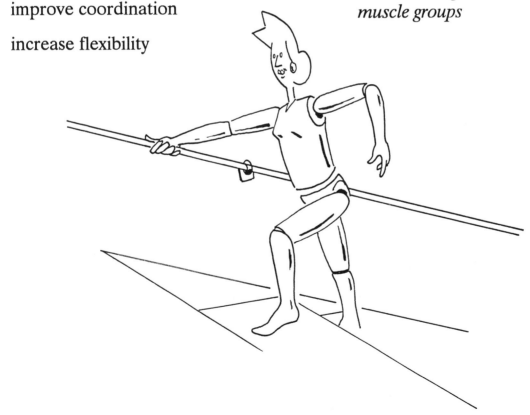

- always have an adequate warm-up period (see ch. 8)

- gradually increase the level (difficulty and intensity) of exercises

- be aware of your breathing when you exercise (don't forget to breathe!)

- watch out for excessive muscle fatigue

- try to do exercises for all of the muscles of the body

- always have an adequate cool-down period (see ch. 8)

DO NOT:

- do not do exercises which involve quick, sharp movements ie. ballistic exercises

- do not do exercises which require a lot of strength

- do not do prolonged strength exercises, e.g. *isometric exercises*

- do not do exercises which overstretch the muscles

- do not do too many repetitions of one exercise (see Chapter 8)

- never bounce when doing stretching exercises

Warning signs of excessive exercise

Stop exercising when:

- you notice a lack of coordination

- you feel:
  a loss of balance

  overfatigued

  muscle soreness

  muscle cramps

  muscle stiffness

Section 5

YOUR LUNGS
(THE RESPIRATORY SYSTEM)

What is the respiratory system ?

- the respiratory system consists of the nose, mouth, throat, *windpipe*, chest muscles, *diaphragm* and lungs

What does it do ?

- it carries oxygen into your body when you breathe in (inhalation)

- it carries carbon dioxide from inside your body to the outside when you breathe out (exhalation)

- it helps protect your body against germs and dust in the air

How does this happen ?

- when you inhale, the ribs, chest muscles and diaphragm help expand the chest cavity and fill the lungs with air (oxygen)

- when you exhale, the ribs, chest muscles and diaphragm help contract the chest cavity to expel air (carbon dioxide) from the lungs

- there are protective parts in the lungs, nose and windpipe which filter germs and dust from the air

In the respiratory system...

aging causes:

- a decrease in the elasticity of the lungs

- a decrease in the ability to absorb oxygen and to get rid of carbon dioxide

- the chest, ribs and diaphragm to become stiffer

- a decrease in the strength of the breathing muscles

- the lungs to become more prone to infection

... so you may notice:

- shallower breathing

- faster breathing

- wheezing

- a shortness of breath

- an increase in *fatigue*

What regular exercise may do for you:

- improve or maintain the elasticity of the lungs, chest, ribs and diaphragm

- improve the circulation of air in the lungs

- strengthen the breathing muscles

- improve overall breathing

Things to remember when you exercise:

- be aware of your breathing when you exercise

- always exercise at your own pace (don't overdo it!)

- try to exercise with a partner and perform the talk test (if you can't keep up a conversation, you're exercising too hard!)

- slow down if you start to cough or breathe heavily

- always exercise in a room which has good air circulation

- wear loose-fitting clothes when you exercise (see ch. 4)

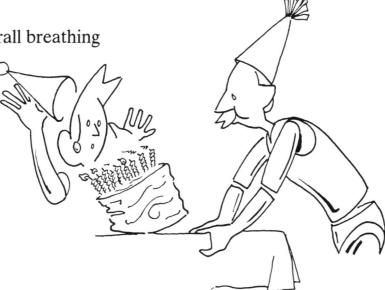

DO NOT:

- do not hold your breath when you exercise (Valsalva manoeuvre)

- never immediately sit down if you are tired (always cool down first or you may faint)

- do not perform exercises which restrict the movement of the chest or abdomen, e.g. exercises done lying on your stomach

- never smoke either immediately before or after exercising (increases heart rate)

Warning signs of excessive exercise

Stop exercising when:

- you find that you cannot talk

- you feel dizzy or lose your balance

- you notice that your skin turns pale

- you cough or wheeze persistently

- you feel excessive fatigue

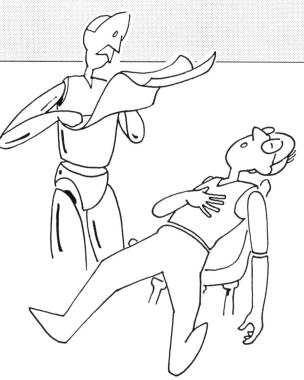

Section 6

YOUR STOMACH AND INTESTINES
(THE DIGESTIVE SYSTEM)

What is the digestive system ?

- the digestive system consists of the mouth, stomach, *intestines* and *rectum*

What does it do ?

- it breaks down the food we eat into smaller pieces

- it absorbs the nutrients after the food is broken down

- it is responsible for the *excretion* of solid body wastes

How does this happen ?

- food is broken down by chewing with the mouth and teeth

- it is digested further in the stomach and intestines through mixing with *acids* and *enzymes*

- the digested food is then absorbed from the intestines into the blood

- body wastes are excreted through the rectum using muscle contractions

In the digestive system...

aging causes:

- an increase in tooth decay

- a decrease in the amount of saliva

- a decrease in chewing ability

- an increase in gum recession

- a drying of the mouth

- a decrease in the sense of taste

- a decrease in the sense of smell

- a decrease in the amount of *mucous* throughout the digestive system

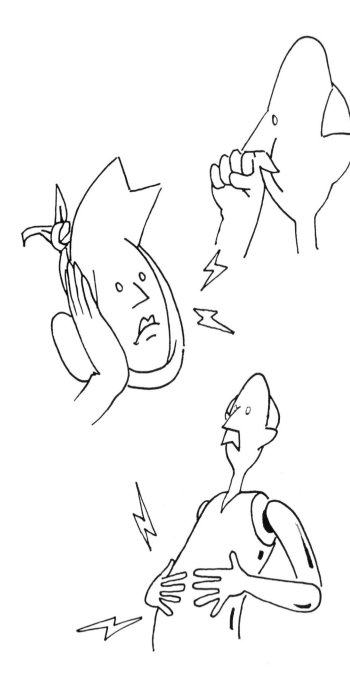

- a decrease in the control of muscles of the digestive system

- a decrease in the amount of acid in the stomach

- a decrease in the secretion of enzymes

- a decrease in the absorption of nutrients

- a decrease in blood flow to the intestines

- an increase in the possibility of bleeding in the stomach or intestines

- a weakening of the rectal muscles

...so you may notice:

- more frequent toothaches

- a difficulty in chewing

- a feeling of discomfort during and after meals

- an increase in the incidence of ulcers

- more frequent burping and passing of gas

- more frequent heartburn

- a difficulty in swallowing

- a loss of appetite

- an increase in the incidence of diarrhea and constipation

- a decrease in the control of the rectum

What regular exercise may do for you:

- increase appetite

- improve the digestive process

- help relieve constipation

Things to remember when you exercise:

- do facial and mouth exercises

- drink water (in moderation) before, during and after exercise

- use the washroom whenever needed during exercising

- relax if excessive burping or heartburn occurs

DO NOT:

- do not eat before, during or immediately following exercise

- do no drink too much liquid before, during or after exercising

- do not drink anything other than water before, during or after exercising

- do not exercise if you feel digestive discomfort

- do not exercise if you have diarrhea

Warning signs of excessive exercise

Stop exercising when:

- you notice a loss of balance

- you experience nausea or vomiting

- you feel heartburn

Section 7

YOUR SKIN
(THE INTEGUMENTARY SYSTEM)

What is the integumentary system ?

- the integumentary system consists of layers of tissue (the skin) that cover the body

What does it do ?

- it provides protection from the environment

- it helps to control your body temperature using *sweat glands*

- it enables you to feel heat, cold, touch and pain

How does this happen ?

- the skin provides protection from the environment by keeping unwanted *particles* and objects out of the body

- protective cells of the skin guard against *bacteria* and *viruses*

- the skin controls your body temperature by opening and closing the *pores* of the skin

- there are specialized cells in the skin which enable you to feel heat, cold, touch and pain

In the integumentary system...

aging causes:

- thinning of the skin

- a decrease in the elasticity of the skin

- roughening of the skin

- a decrease in the amount of *skin pigment*

- dryness of the skin

- a decrease in blood flow to the skin

- a decrease in the ability to replace skin cells

- a decrease in the number of sweat glands

- a decrease in the number of specialized cells

... so you may notice:

- a decrease in the healing ability of the skin, e.g. bruises

- wrinkles

- paleness of the skin

- a progressively increasing number of brown spots

- a decrease in the control of body temperature

- a decreased resistance to sunburning

What regular exercise may do for you:

- increase the flow of blood to the skin

- maintain the number and function of sweat glands

- moisten the skin

- slow down the roughening of the skin

- slow down the drying of the skin

- slow down the loss of skin pigments

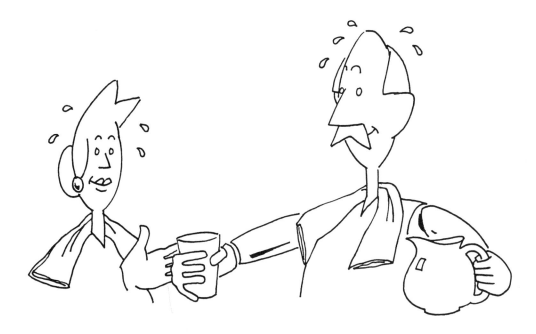

Things to remember when you exercise:

- make sure that the room is at a comfortable exercising temperature

- wear clothes that 'breathe' (see ch. 4)

- always wear proper footwear (see ch. 4)

- wear clothes that are not rough on the skin

- do floor exercises on carpets, mats or towels

- wear cotton socks rather than nylons

DO NOT:
- do not perform exercises that rub the skin on the floor

- do not perform exercises on rough surfaces

- do not exercise wearing improper footwear

- do not exercise wearing jewellery

REFERENCES

Bourne, G. H. (Ed.). (1967). Endocrines and aging. Springfield: Charles C Thomas.

Garn, S. M. (Ed.). (1975). The physiology and pathology of human aging. New York: Academic Press.

Graham, R. (Ed.). (1973). Textbook of geriatric medicine and gerontology. London: Churchill Livingstone.

Han, S. S., & Coons, D.H. (Eds.). (1979). Special senses in aging. Michigan: Ann Arbor.

Rossman, I. (1979). Clinical geriatrics (2nd ed.). Philadelphia: Lippincott.

Shephard, R. J. (1978). Physical activity and aging (2nd ed.). Kent: Croom Helm.

Smith, E. L., & Serfass, R. C. (Eds.). (1981). Exercise and aging: The scientific basis. New Jersey: Enslow.

Timiras, P. S. (Ed.). (1988). Physiological basis of geriatrics. New York: Macmillan.

CHAPTER 2

COMMON PHYSICAL DISORDERS

This chapter deals with a variety of common physical *disorders* of the elderly on which regular exercise can have a positive effect. The disorders discussed in this chapter include *arthritis*, *osteoporosis*, problems with the heart and circulatory system, and *maturity-onset diabetes*.

Unfortunately, misinformation and lack of knowledge have led to many misconceptions about these conditions. The intent of this chapter is to provide you with a better understanding of these disorders, their possible causes and methods for improving and/or preventing them.

Remember, the suggestions presented in this chapter are to be meant for your information only and must not take the place of your physician's advice.

The disorders discussed herein are all serious conditions. Any treatment from any source should be used with caution, common sense and only with the approval of your physician.

Section 1

ARTHRITIS

There are over 100 types of arthritis. Each type of arthritis is different, therefore, needs different treatment. Arthritis may cause pain, stiffness, swelling, tenderness or *inflammation* of the joints or affected areas. It can also prevent some movements which are necessary for the activities of daily living.

It is important that people should try to learn as much as possible about this *disease* so that they may be able to understand how to control it.

Did you know that:

- arthritis affects people from all age groups

- arthritis cannot be cured but may be controlled

- arthritis is a disease which usually lasts a lifetime but, in many cases, there are periods in which few or no symptoms are apparent (periods of *remission*)

- arthritis means that you have changes in one or more of the following parts of your joint(s):

Functional Parts of a Joint:

Cartilage:
A tough material that cushions and protects the ends of bones. (Example of arthritis in this part: osteoarthritis.)

Synovial Membrane:
A thin layer of tissue which surrounds the joint and contains and produces a *lubricating fluid* (synovial fluid). This fluid oils the joint and is also responsible for keeping the cartilage healthy. (Examples of arthritis in this part: rheumatoid arthritis, gout.)

Bursa:
A small sac located near the joint which contains a lubricating fluid. This sac allows smooth movement of

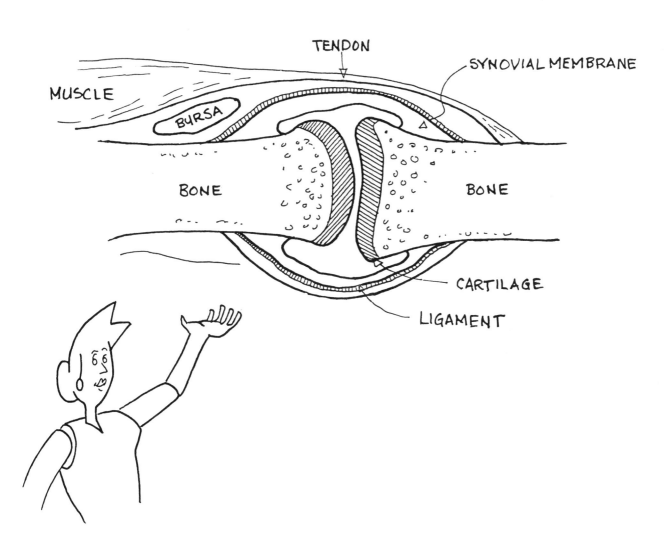

muscle across muscle and tendon across bone. (Example of inflammation in this part: bursitis.)

Muscle:
The muscles are elastic tissues that work together to move the bones by contracting and relaxing. (Example of involvement of this part: fibrositis.)

Tendon:
Tissue fibre which attaches muscle to bone. (Example of involvement of this part: tendonitis.)

Ligament:
Tissue fibre which attaches bone to bone. (Example of arthritis in this part: ankylosing spondylitis.)

Since there are so many different types of arthritis, only two forms will be discussed in this section. These are: *osteoarthritis*, and *rheumatoid arthritis*, the two most common forms.

OSTEOARTHRITIS

Also called:

> *Degenerative* joint disease

> Degenerative arthritis

> Osteoarthrosis

What is it ?

Osteoarthritis is a degenerative disease which most often affects the 'weight-bearing joints', i.e. ankles, knees, hips, spine. The cartilage breaks down, tears or rips, and leaves the bone surfaces without a cushion.

How do I get it ?

The cause of osteoarthritis is not definitely known, but it can be caused by one or more of the following factors:

- normal wear and tear

- injuries to joints

- the natural aging process

- heredity

- abuse of joints

- insufficient use of joints

How does it affect me ?

The tears or rips may cause the joint to 'catch' or 'lock'.

Bony growths of 'spurs' may appear in the affected joint, causing intense pain and limited movement.

Due to the lack of cartilage, bone surfaces rub together resulting in pain and limited movement.

What can I do ?

1. See your physician: your physician knows both you and your disease, and can recommend a treatment that is best for you.

2. Exercise: if performed correctly and on a regular basis, exercises help maintain and can improve body movements and functions.

3. Control weight: maintaining your ideal weight will minimize stress on your joints.

4. Stay active: regular use of joints is important to keep them healthy and strong.

5. Use heat/cold treatments: heat and/or cold treatments may help reduce joint pain and swelling.

6. Use special devices: special devices may help a person with their day-to-day living, e.g. extended handles on brushes, mops, brooms, etc., objects to help dress yourself such as button threaders, canes, crutches, walkers.

7. Inform yourself: find out as much about this disease as you can!

Always consult with your physician before attempting any self treatment program !

RHEUMATOID ARTHRITIS

What is it ?

Rheumatoid arthritis is a *disorder* which involves many of the body's systems and often affects the toes, ankles, knees, shoulders, elbows and fingers. The synovial membrane, which lines the joint, becomes inflamed. About one person in 100 of the population have rheumatoid arthritis, and two to three times more women do than men.

How do I get it ?

There is no known specific cause of rheumatoid arthritis, but the latest theories suggest that it develops from a viral or *bacterial infection.*

It is an *auto-immune* disease, which means your body is attacked by its own defence system.

How does it affect me ?

Rheumatoid arthritis causes many problems because it works on many of the body's systems.

Some of these problems are:

- pain
- swelling
- weakness
- fatigue
- stiffness
- weight loss
- fever
- joint deformity

What can I do ?

1. See your physician: your physician knows both you and your disease, and can recommend a treatment that is best for you.

2. Exercise: if performed correctly and regularly, exercise may help maintain or increase the range of motion and stability of the affected joints.

3. Stay active: if a person sits for a long period of time, joints may become stiff and painful to move.

4. Rest: *fatigue* is common in rheumatoid arthritis, therefore rest is needed regularly in order to reduce inflammation.

5. Use heat/cold treatments: heat and/or cold treatments may help reduce joint pain and swelling.

6. Use special devices: special devices may help a person with day-to-day living, e.g. extended handles on brushes, mops, brooms, etc., objects to help dress yourself such as button threaders, canes, crutches, walkers.

7. Inform yourself: find out as much about this disease as you can!

Always consult with your physician before attempting any self treatment program !

What should I know before I exercise with arthritis ?

Always consult with your physician before doing any physcial activity!

1. Exercise carefully on a regular basis and at a slow pace to build range of motion and muscle strength.

2. Do not overstrain yourself. Your guide to knowing whether or not you have exercised too much is pain.

3. Exercising should be done in a gradual progression — always exercise your worst joints first.

4. Do not exercise a joint if it is inflamed.

5 . To relieve stress on your spine, lie flat on your back, arms at sides, feet slightly apart.

6. Avoid quick or sharp movments when exercising (ballistic exercises).

7. Avoid jumping while exercising.

8. Be sure to share all information on any medical problems you may have with **ALL** physicians who work with you. They need to know as much as possible about you and your body to help you in the best way possible.

Section 2

OSTEOPOROSIS

Osteoporosis is a common condition affecting the older population, and in advanced cases may cause severe crippling. When a person has osteoporosis, their bones become brittle due to bone loss and, as a result, may *fracture* quite easily.

Early signs of osteoporosis, affecting close to one million Canadian women, are rather vague or completely lacking until a fracture occurs. Loss of height and the beginning of 'dowager's hump', along with back pain, would be sufficient warning to request evaluation. Men are not exempt, especially if they are of small stature, suffer from overuse of alcohol and tobacco, are on certain medications, or have reached 70 years of age. Males are usually affected at a later age simply because they have a greater bone density to start with (as do blacks). Normal loss of bone density for males occurs at a slower and steadier rate than for females. During the first five years of menopause in women, studies show that the rate of bone loss can be six times that of men. Around the age of 65 to 70, it slows down again to a rate more equal to that of men.

It is important that people should try to learn as much as possible about this disorder so that they may be able to help prevent it and understand how to control it.

Did you know that?:

- some degree of osteoporosis occurs in about two-thirds of women over 65 years of age, but only in about one-fifth of men

- with the normal aging process, *bone mass* decreases faster than it can replace itself, resulting in a gradual loss of bone density

Recent statistics state that osteoporosis is so widespread it has already reached epidemic proportions and is placing enormous costs on the health care system.

What is it ?

Osteoporosis (porous bone) is a loss of bone mass or density. It is a silent thief that starts when you are younger and manifests itself when you are older. It is a condition by which the pores of bone gradually become enlarged (holey bones), thus weakening the structure, until one day, a fracture occurs from some trivial incident, such as a good sneeze or hug or a minor fall. An x-ray confirms the fracture, but osteoporosis cannot be detected unless 30 to 35% of bone density is already lost. Osteoporotic bone differs in no way from normal bone, there is just less of it.

How do I get it ?

If you fit into one or more of these categories, you are at a higher risk of having osteoporosis, and you should see your physician:

- you are a *post-menopausal* female

- you are of North European or Asian descent

- you are small framed

- you are light boned

- you have a slim figure

- you lack calcium in your diet

- you lead an inactive (sedentary) lifestyle

- your family has a history of osteoporosis

- you smoke, drink, or use drugs excessively

- your doctor has determined that you have a *hormone deficiency*

- you have been diagnosed as having hyperparathyroidism

- your ovaries have been surgically removed

- you have never been pregnant

How does it affect me ?

It may cause joint pain.

In osteoporosis, the *vertebrae* become brittle and in severe cases can collapse from the body's weight.

This may cause:

- a *deformed* spine or humped back (dowager's hump)

- chronic back pain

- loss of several inches in height

In severe cases, it may cause bones to fracture easily for no apparent reason, even while turning in bed.

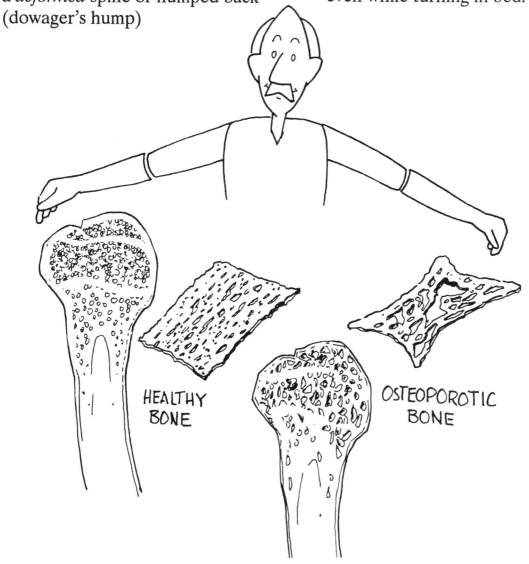

HEALTHY BONE

OSTEOPOROTIC BONE

What can I do ?

1. See your physician: your physician knows both you and your disease, and can recommend a treatment that is best for you.

2. Exercise regularly (weight-bearing exercises as opposed to water exercises): exercising properly and staying active will help strengthen bones.

3. Eat nutritious meals and a balanced diet; make sure that daily requirements of calcium and vitamin D are met. This may help rebuild bones.

4. Stop or decrease tobacco, coffee or alcohol intake.

> **Always consult with your physician before attempting any self treatment program!**

What should I know before I exercise with osteoporosis ?

It has been said that exercise is the only preventive and therapeutic measure that not only halts bone loss, but also stimulates the formation of new bone. (Bone is like muscle - use it or lose it.)

When preparing to participate in a physical activity program the following guidelines are offered:

> **Always consult with your physician before doing any physical activity!**

1. Choose a program for both the upper and lower extremities.

2. A 20 minute brisk walk daily, preferably in the sunshine for Vitamin D benefits, is an easy and effective weight-bearing exercise.

3. Exercise on a regular basis for maximum benefit (approximately three times per week).

4. A good way to avoid/relieve stress on the spine when exercising is to lie flat on your back (when possible), arms at sides, with knees bent until feet are flat on the floor and slightly apart.

5. Avoid exercising with weights unless medically approved.

6. Avoid sudden or sharp movements or jumping forms of exercises.

7. Be sure to share all information on any medical problems you may have with <u>ALL</u> physicians who work with you. They need to know as much as possible about you and your body to help you in the best way possible.

Exercising without following the above precautions may result in strain, pain or fractures in people with osteoporosis in any physical fitness program.

Section 3

PROBLEMS WITH THE HEART AND CIRCULATORY SYSTEM

Your heart is a hollow muscle, about the size of your fist, located in the centre of your chest and tilted slightly to the left. Like a pump, the heart's role is to circulate blood throughout the body through the *arteries* and *veins*.

The heart is the most important muscle in the body and affects many of the body's functions, therefore when your heart does not function properly, your whole body becomes less efficient.

It is important to learn as much as possible about how some types of heart and circulatory problems may be avoided or controlled so that you can prevent it from happening to you or someone you know.

Did you know that:

- heart disease is the number one killer in North America

- the average resting heart rate is approximately 50 to 100 beats per minute, over 100,000 times a day and approximately 2.5 billion times in a lifetime; this resting heart rate decreases as we age

- the heart pumps approximately five litres of blood to the body every minute at rest, and approximately 30 to 35 litres per minute when exercising

- your blood vessels stretched end to end could circle the earth twice

In this section, we will talk about:

- high blood pressure
- *arteriosclerosis*
- *atherosclerosis*
- *congestive heart failure*
- *aneurysm*
- *stroke*
- angina
- heart attack

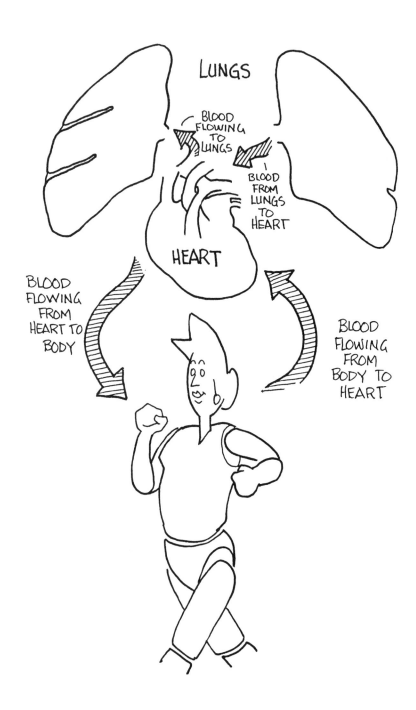

HIGH BLOOD PRESSURE

Also called:

- Hypertension

What is blood pressure ?

When your heart beats, blood is forced through your elastic-like arteries, causing them to expand. When your heart is resting between beats, your arteries relax and return to their original shape. The force of blood against the artery walls is called blood pressure.

When your physician takes your blood pressure, he is actually recording two different measurements. The first measurement, which is always the higher of the two, measures the force against the artery walls when the heart is pumping and the arteries are expanding (systolic pressure). The second measurement is the pressure exerted when your heart and arteries are relaxed (diastolic pressure). An example of a blood pressure reading would be 120/80, with 120 being the systolic pressure, and 80 being the diastolic pressure.

What is high blood pressure ?

High blood pressure is a condition in which the blood pressure is too high and remains above the normal limits. This can lead to many other problems.

How do I get it ?

High blood pressure is not a condition which suddenly occurs. There are many contributing factors which may lead to high blood pressure. These are:

- family history of high blood pressure

- inactive lifestyle

- obesity

- aging

- excessive sodium (salt) or fat intake

- stressful lifestyle

- excessive alcohol or tobacco consumption

- gender — a higher percentage of males suffer from this condition

- race — blacks are more susceptible than whites

- kidney problems

How does it affect me ?

If you have high blood pressure, you may not even know it. High blood pressure is called a 'silent disease' meaning that there are no obvious symptoms; however, if left untreated, high blood pressure may lead to:

- heart attack

- stroke

- kidney trouble

- other heart or circulatory problems

ATHEROSCLEROSIS

What is it ?

Atherosclerosis is a build up of fatty deposits (such as *cholesterol*) in the arteries. The arteries become clogged and narrow, preventing blood from flowing properly through your body. This vascular disease may lead to many other problems.

How do I get it ?

The three major contributors to atherosclerosis are believed to be:

- high cholesterol level in the blood

- smoking

- high blood pressure

How does it affect me ?

Atherosclerosis causes the heart to have to work harder to pump the blood through the arteries. You may not experience any symptoms because sometimes when an artery is clogged, other blood vessels may take over for a period of time. This extra work forced upon the heart may lead to:

- stroke

- heart attack

- high blood pressure

- aneurysm (due to weakened arterial walls)

- other heart or circulatory problems

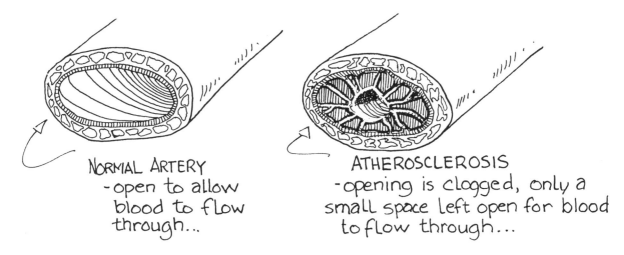

NORMAL ARTERY
-open to allow
blood to flow
through...

ATHEROSCLEROSIS
-opening is clogged, only a
small space left open for blood
to flow through...

ARTERIOSCLEROSIS

Also called:

- Hardening of the arteries

What is it ?

Arteriosclerosis is a disease which causes the artery walls to thicken and lose their elasticity. This prevents blood from flowing properly through your body, placing more stress on the heart. This may lead to many other heart or circulatory problems.

How do I get it ?

Arteriosclerosis is thought to be caused by:

- the normal aging process

- excessive smoking

How does it affect me ?

Arteriosclerosis causes the heart to have to work harder to pump the blood through the arteries. There may be no obvious symptoms of arteriosclerosis; however, if left untreated, this extra work forced upon the heart may lead to:

- stroke

- heart attack

- angina

- high blood pressure

- other heart or circulatory problems

CONGESTIVE HEART FAILURE

What is it ?

Congestive heart failure is a condition in which the heart becomes weak and unable to pump enough blood to meet the needs of the body. This causes the *blood circulation* to slow down and become inefficient.

How do I get it ?

There are two main factors which are known to cause the heart to weaken. These two factors are:

- the results of other heart problems, e.g. heart attack

- high blood pressure

How does it affect me ?

Congestive heart failure may cause fluid to pool in your body especially in the extremities (hands and feet) and lungs. Congestive heart failure may also cause:

- swollen ankles

- swollen abdomen

- difficulty in breathing (not only when exercising)

- chest pains

- loss of appetite

- nausea

- reduced amount of urine

- dry cough

- accelerated heart rate

- decrease in blood pressure

- irregular heart beat (palpitations)

- drowsiness, confusion, loss of concentration

ANEURYSM

What is it ?

An aneurysm is a weakened segment of an artery or other blood vessel that fills with blood and balloons outward much like a bulging weak spot in an inflated tire inner tube.

How do I get it ?

An aneurysm may be caused by:

- atherosclerosis

- high blood pressure

- defect present from birth

How does it affect me ?

If an aneurysm ruptures (breaks), it may cause:

- stroke

- internal bleeding

- unconsciousness

- severe headaches

- muscle weakness

- death

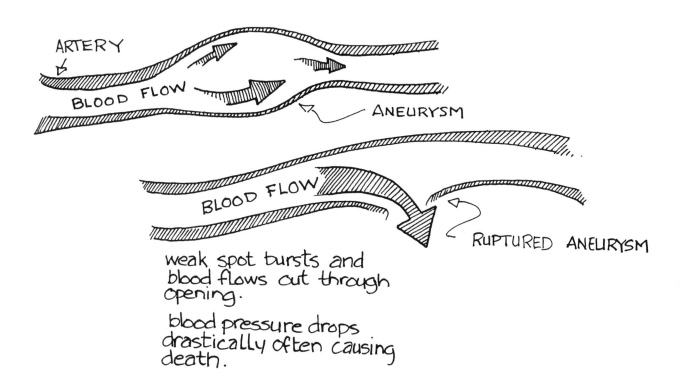

ARTERY

BLOOD FLOW

ANEURYSM

BLOOD FLOW

RUPTURED ANEURYSM

weak spot bursts and blood flows out through opening.

blood pressure drops drastically often causing death.

STROKE

Also called:
- Cerebrovascular accident (CVA)

What is it ?

A stroke occurs when there is a lack of oxygen and blood flow to a part of the brain due to a problem with the circulation of blood to this part. This may be due to a *blood clot*, aneurysm, head injury (cerebral haemorrhage) or other obstruction in an artery. A stroke usually results in the death of the affected area of the brain.

How do I get it ?

Some of the factors which may contribute to the risk of stroke are:
- atherosclerosis
- high blood pressure
- blood clots
- aneurysms
- aging
- obesity
- history of 'mini-strokes' *
- family history of strokes
- race — Negroes are more susceptable that whites
- excessive smoking
- *diabetes*
- inactive or sedentary lifestyle

*Mini-strokes (transient ischaemic attacks) are usually a warning of a major stroke. They occur when the flow of blood to the brain is momentarily blocked or diminished. A person experiencing a mini-stroke may have a brief dizzy spell, a feeling of confusion, temporary clumsiness, an increase in the number and severity of headaches, or a noticeable change in personality. Mini-strokes only affect a small portion of the brain so you may be only slightly aware that something is wrong. If you experience these symptoms and they continue or become worse, you should contact your physician.

How does it affect me ?

Depending on the area of the brain that is affected, a stroke may cause:

- paralysis

- loss of one or more senses

- speech problems

- vision impairments

- loss of memory

- change in personality

- change in mental ability

- *aphasia*

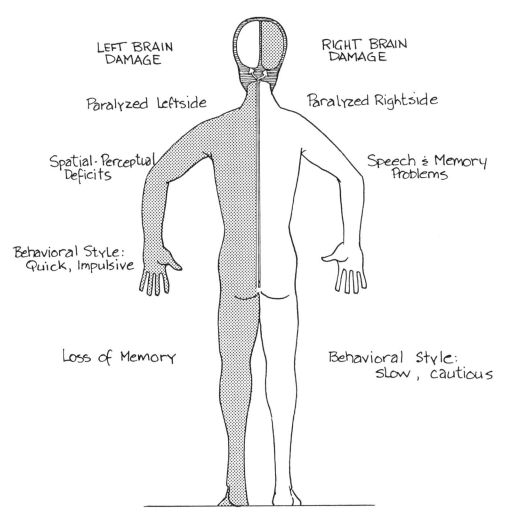

AFFECTS OF A STROKE...

LEFT BRAIN DAMAGE

RIGHT BRAIN DAMAGE

Paralyzed Leftside

Paralyzed Rightside

Spatial-Perceptual Deficits

Speech & Memory Problems

Behavioral Style: Quick, Impulsive

Loss of Memory

Behavioral Style: slow, cautious

How do I know if I am having a stroke?

The signs of a stroke include one or more of the following symptoms:

- sudden weakness or numbness of the face, arm or leg on one side of the body.

- loss of speech, trouble speaking or understanding speech

- unexplained dizziness, unsteadiness or sudden falls

- dimmed vision, loss of vision or double vision in one eye

What should I do if I am having a stroke ?

Get help immediately!

1. Call for emergency help or summon a person close by when symptoms begin.

2. Stop activity and sit or lie down.

3. Do not take any food or drink.

4. Loosen clothing.

5. Try to remain as calm as possible — do not panic.

What should I do if I am with somebody who is having a stroke ?

Act immediately!

1. Take charge and give reassurance — the victim will likely deny what is happening.

2. Call an emergency rescue service or go to the nearest hospital emergency room.

3. Have the victim stop activity and help them into a sitting or lying position.

4. Loosen clothing.

5. DO NOT give the person anything to eat or drink.

ANGINA PECTORIS

Angina is not a heart attack.

What is it ?

Angina is a passing (temporary), dull pain felt in the chest due to part of the heart demanding more blood and oxygen than is actually being supplied. If this deficiency is not too great, angina is the result. If the deficiency is too great, a heart attack may be the result.

How do I get it ?

Factors which contribute to angina are similar to those of other heart problems which cause the heart to overwork. Some of these are:

- physical or emotional stress
- excessive smoking
- high cholesterol level in the blood
- high blood pressure

How does it affect me ?

Angina may cause you to feel:

- a dull, pressing or constricting pain in the chest
- heaviness, tightness, burning pressure or squeezing sensation in the chest
- breathlessness during activity

HEART ATTACK

Also called:
- myocardial infarction
- coronary thrombosis

What is it ?

A heart attack occurs when there is a blockage (usually a blood clot) in an artery which supplies blood to a part of the heart muscle. This part is starved of nutrients and oxygen and it begins to die.

When a heart attack occurs...

Within one minute, the area of the heart deprived of oxygen and blood fatigues then beats rapidly (fibrillations) and within four minutes that part dies.

How do I get it ?

There are many factors which lead to heart attacks. The more contributing factors you have, the higher the risk of heart attack. Some of these factors are:
- lack of exercise
- high blood pressure
- smoking
- stressful lifestyle
- high cholesterol level in the blood
- family history of heart attacks
- obesity

How does it affect me ?

A heart attack will affect different people in different ways and may have many long lasting physical and/or psychological effects such as increased risk of congestive heart failure, recurring heart attacks or fear of death.

How do I know if I am having a heart attack ?

The signs of a heart attack include one or more of the following symptoms:
- prolonged, heavy, squeezing pain or discomfort in the centre of the chest (sometimes mistaken for *indigestion*)
- pain in the neck, jaw, arms, upper abdomen and / or between the shoulder blades

- severe pain, dizziness, fainting, sweating, nausea, shortness of breath, anxiety and/or greyish skin colour may also occur

What should I do if I am having a heart attack?

Get help immediately!

1. Call for emergency help or, if able, summon a person close by.

2. Sit in a half-lying, half-sitting position.

3. Do not take any food or drink.

4. Loosen clothing.

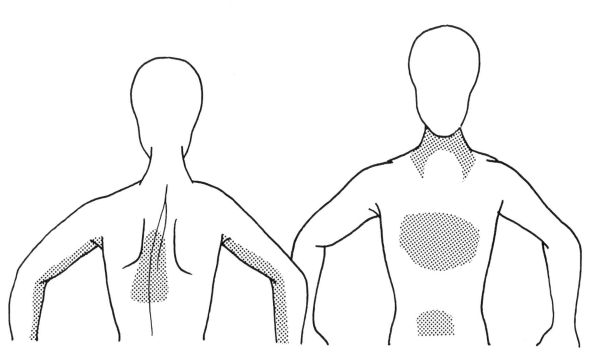

WARNING SIGNS OF A HEART ATTACK
Shaded areas indicate painful areas during a heart attack.

5. Try to remain as calm as possible — do not panic.

What should I do if I'm with somebody who is having a heart attack ?

Act immediately

If you are qualified: give *cardiopulmonary resuscitation (CPR)*. **(CPR is a life-saving technique usually used to help victims of choking or heart attacks.)**

1. Take charge and give reassurance — the victim will likely deny what is happening.

2. Call an emergency rescue service, or go to the nearest hospital emergency room.

3. Have the victim stop activity and put them in a half-sitting, half-lying position.

4. Loosen clothing.

5. Ask the victim if they have been prescribed any emergency heart medication (e.g. nitroglycerine), if so, help with administering medication.

6. DO NOT give the person anything to eat or drink.

What can I do to prevent or control heart or circulatory problems ?

1. Consult your physician: your physician is familiar with both you and your condition. He may be able to prescribe a treatment which best suits your needs.

2. Exercise: if performed correctly and regularly, exercise will strengthen your heart and arteries. Losing excess weight will also reduce excess strain on your heart.

3. Proper diet: eating well-balanced meals (low in salt and saturated fats) may reduce the risks of high blood pressure and build up of cholesterol, which are the main contributors to other heart or circulatory problems.

3. Quit smoking: smoking is very harmful to your heart and arteries. Smoking causes the heart to beat more rapidly and decreases the amount of oxygen in your blood. Quitting this habit reduces the risk of heart or circulatory problems.

4. Limit alcohol: alcohol may raise blood pressure causing your heart to work harder. Alcohol should be taken in moderation.

5. Control stress: stress cannot always be avoided; learning to relax and get plenty of rest and sleep will prove beneficial. Enjoy life and have fun!

> **Always consult with your physician before attempting <u>any</u> self treatment program!**

What should I know before exercising with heart or circulatory problems ?

> **Always consult with your physician before doing any physical activity!**

1. Exercise on a regular basis, at a slow pace and with gradual progression.

2. Do not overstrain yourself.

3. If you feel fatigued or experience pain, dizziness or shortness of breath, stop exercising immediately.

4. Do not overdo it! If your body tells you to stop, then stop!

5. Be sure to share all information on any medical problems you may have with <u>ALL</u> physicians that work with you. They need to know as much as possible about you and your body to help you in the best way possible.

Why should I be careful when exercising with heart or circulatory problems ?

A heart condition should not be taken lightly. Exercising at the same rate as a person with a healthy heart may further damage your heart.

There are various degrees of stroke which affect people in different ways. You should always consult your physician for the exercises that are appropriate for your rehabilitation.

Section 4

DIABETES

Diabetes is a condition in which your body can not properly use or control the amount of sugar (*glucose*) in your blood. The primary cause of diabetes is inadequate production or inefficient use of *insulin*.

Insulin is produced by the *pancreas*, a gland located behind the stomach. Insulin is a *hormone* which is essential to the conversion of the food (sugar) that we eat into energy.

In a diabetic, either the pancreas or the process of changing sugar into energy does not function properly. The result of this malfunction is a high glucose level in the blood.

If not controlled, diabetes may result in serious consequences. In order to control your diabetes, you must learn about it so that you are able to continue a normal lifestyle.

Did you know that:

- diabetes is the single most frequent reason for visits to the doctor and hospitalization

- approximately one-half of people with some form of diabetes do not know they have it

- an untreated severe diabetic loses the equivalent of approximately 247 kg (545 lbs.) of sugar in the urine every year

There are two main types of diabetes. In type I or insulin dependant diabetes (*juvenile diabetes*), the pancreas does not produce insulin. In type II or non-insulin dependant diabetes (maturity-onset diabetes), an adequate amount of insulin is produced but is not properly used.

In the following section, we will discuss maturity-onset diabetes only, since the aging process plays a major role in the onset of this type of diabetes.

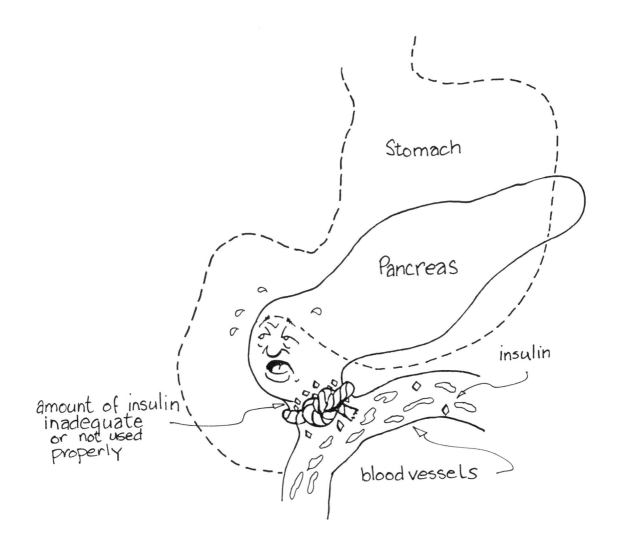

MATURITY-ONSET DIABETES

Also called:

- Type II diabetes

- Non-insulin dependant diabetes

What is it ?

Maturity-onset diabetes is a disease which is found more commonly in people over forty. The body produces an adequate amount of insulin, but cannot use it properly.

How do I get it ?

Factors which contribute to the risk of maturity-onset diabetes are:

- obesity
- family history of maturity-onset diabetes
- age (over 40)
- stress (physical or emotional)
- inactivity
- poor diet

How does it affect me ?

If maturity-onset diabetes is not monitored and controlled, it may lead to serious consequences such as:

- stroke
- heart problems
- nerve damage
- kidney failure
- *gangrene*
- foot problems
- vision problems
- skin infections
- seizures or coma

What can I do ?

1. See your physician: your physician knows both you and your condition, and can recommend a treatment that is best for you.

2. Exercise regularly: exercising properly and staying active will help reduce or maintain weight and help control your blood sugar, decreasing the risks of diabetes.

3. Eat a balanced diet: eat nutritious meals and a balanced diet, making sure that your diabetic menu is followed.

4. Inform yourself: find out as much about this condition as you can! The more you know, the better you will understand what is happening to your body.

5. Monitor your condition: keep your blood sugar within the accepted level. Work with your physician to determine the best way to ensure correct sugar levels, i.e. urine testing, insulin injections, medication.

Always consult with your physician before attempting <u>any</u> self-treatment program!

What should I know before exercising with maturity-onset diabetes ?

Always consult with your physician before doing any physical activity!

1. Exercise on a regular basis, at a slow pace and with gradual progression.

2. Do not overstrain yourself.

3. Be sure to eat proper food before exercising. Do not exercise on an empty stomach.

4. Be sure to share all information on any medical problems you may have with <u>ALL</u> physicians that work with you. They need to know as much as possible about you and your body to help you in the best way possible.

Why should I be careful when exercising with maturity-onset diabetes ?

Physical activity can alter your blood sugar level. Be aware of how you feel before, during and after physical activity. If you begin to experience weakness, dizziness, abdominal pain, nausea, headache, blurred vision, shaking or trembling, then STOP ! If these feelings persist after rest:

- administer insulin if this is your normal procedure

- contact your physician

- if these symptoms continue and/or become worse, get help immediately and go to the nearest hospital

REFERENCES

Baker, P. (1983). Coping with arthritis. Richmond Hill, Ontario: Irwin.

Cooley, D. G. (Ed.). (1987). Family medical guide. New York: Meredith Corporation.

Guiness, A. (Ed.). (1987). ABC's of the human body. Pleasantville, New York: Reader's Digest Association.

Hegele, R.A. (1989). Like father, like son: The genetic factor in heart disease. Healthwatch, pp. 31-36.

Keough, C. (Ed.). (1987). Future youth: How to reverse the aging process. Emmaus, Pennsylvania: Rodale Press.

Lorig, K., & Fries, J. (1986). The arthritis help book (rev. ed.). Reading, Massachusetts: Addison-Wesley.

Notelovitz, M., & Ware, M. (1982). Stand tall: Every woman's guide to preventing osteoporosis. Gainsville, Florida: Triad.

Spence, A. P. (1989). Biology of human aging. New Jersey: Prentice-Hall.

Spirduso, W. W., & Eckert, H. M. (Eds.). (1989). Physical activity and aging. Champagne, Illinois: Human Kinetics Books.

Subak-Sharpe, G., & Weiss, R. J. (Eds.). (1988). Complete guide to health and well-being after 50. New York: Random House.

The Canadian Red Cross Society & YWCA. (1986). A fitness leader's guide to osteoporosis. Toronto: Government of Canada.

Wantz, M. S,. & Gay, J. E. (1981). The aging process: A health perspective. Cambridge, Massachusetts: Winthrop.

CHAPTER 3

LIVING WITH AGING

No matter what your age, your body is changing both inside and outside — year by year and day by day. We know that during a baby's first 12 months, the changes that take place are readily apparent. As this first year unfolds, we see a transformation of facial features and physique as well as changes in eating and sleeping habits. Remarkable also is the developing and maturing of communication and learning skills. Changes continue to occur to a lesser degree throughout our entire lifetime — these changes we refer to as 'aging'. When attributing these changes to young people, we call it 'maturing' but when someone reaches middle age, we refer to it as 'aging'. Aging may now take on a negative meaning; it reminds us that we are getting older. Yes, there are changes that occur as we grow older, but this transformation began a long time ago and rather than take a negative attitude toward your maturing body, you should be proud to wear your new look.

The following chapter explains the differences you may notice in your body, both on the outside and inside, and offers you some suggestions to make you comfortable with your maturing body.

SECTION 1

BODY CHANGES AND ATTITUDES

APPEARANCE

Our physical appearance can greatly influence the way we feel about ourselves. It is constantly changing as we age and we become older looking throughout our lives. Changes in appearance in later years can be a source of frustration for some people if they associate such changes with a loss of attractiveness. Fortunately, a lot can be done to maintain a more youthful appearance.

WHAT CHANGES AFFECT MY APPEARANCE?

Many physical changes that occur with age affect one's appearance. You may notice some or all of the following changes:

CHANGES IN BODY SHAPE, HEIGHT & POSTURE

Fat Redistribution

There is a loss of fat from the arms, legs, neck and face, and a gain of fat on the hips and body due to a redistribution of fatty tissue.

Overall Fat Gain

Older persons tend to gain fat in areas where muscle loss has occurred due to aging.

Narrowing of Shoulders, Arms and Legs

Narrowing of these areas results from a loss of muscle with age.

Loss of Height

A decrease in height occurs due to a shortening of weakened bones in the spine and a thinning of cartilage between vertebrae.

Poor Posture

Poor posture results from a curving of the weakened bones in the spine.

SKIN CHANGES

Dry, Wrinkled, Sagging Skin

Dry skin is due to the fact that less oxygen and fewer nutrients reach the skin from the capillaries. There is also a loss of sweat glands and a slower renewal of oil cells as we age. Wrinkled skin occurs because of a loss of elasticity. Sagging skin is due to a loss of fat underneath the skin.

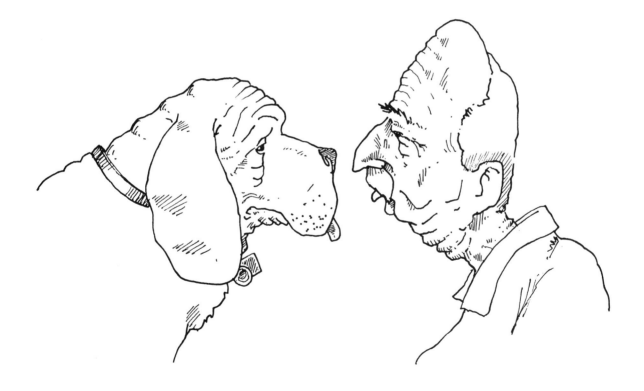

Paleness

Pale skin occurs due to an overall loss of *pigment* cells in the skin.

Age/Liver Spots

These spots result from collections of a certain skin pigment in heavily exposed areas, such as the face and hands.

Prominent Blood Vessels

Blood vessels become more noticeable due to thinning of the skin.

HAIR CHANGES

Hair Loss

Loss of hair on head, arms and pubic area occurs due to the decrease in the number and the productivity of *hair follicles*.

Thickening of Facial Hair

Hair on the face may thicken and grow coarser. In the female, this is due to a reduction in the number of female hormones (estrogen)present. Females begin to take on some male characteristics, e.g. thicker and coarser hair on face, nose, ears and eyebrows.

In the male, changes that may result are loss of hair on head, coarser hair in beard, hair on ears, nose, etc.

Greying

Hair turns grey because of a loss of pigment cells in the hair.

Dryness

Dry hair results from a reduction in the number of oil glands in the scalp.

CHANGES IN FACIAL STRUCTURE

Strong Features

Bonier areas of the face (nose, cheekbones) appear larger due to a loss of fat underneath the skin.

Flatter Nose, Longer Ears

A flattening of the nose and lengthening of the ears occur as a result of thinning cartilage in these areas.

Sagging Areas

Jowls and loose skin on the neck form due to a loss of elasticity of the skin and a loss of fat underneath the skin.

Sunken Cheeks and Eyes

Sunken cheeks and eyes develop from a loss of fat underneath the skin.

NAIL CHANGES

Hard, Brittle Nails

Brittle, hard nails occur due to a thickening of the surface layer of nails.

TEETH CHANGES

Tooth Loss

A loss of one or more teeth is due to a deterioration of the gums, often leading to *periodontal* (gum) diseases.

All of these changes occur at different rates and to different degrees for different people. You may notice one of these changes at 40, or not until past your 80s. However, there are many factors other than aging itself which can age your appearance.

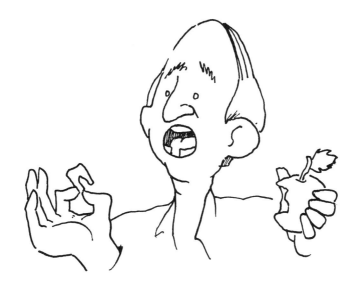

WHAT ELSE AFFECTS MY APPEARANCE?

Heredity

The effect which aging has on our appearance is partly due to heredity. The *genetic* characteristics of your parents were passed on to you and play a large part in determining when and to what extent you will experience changes in appearance with age.

Active/Inactive Lifestyle

An inactive lifestyle leads to further decline in the capacity and *efficiency* of the body's systems. This enhances the aging process and therefore results in a more aged appearance. An active lifestyle however, improves capacity and efficiency of these systems and can slow down or even reverse some of the effects of aging.

Eating Habits

Your appearance reflects how well you nourish your body. (After all, you are what you eat!) Poor eating habits deprive your body of the nourishment you need to keep your body running smoothly and looking healthy.

Drinking and Smoking Habits

Drinking large amounts of alcohol on a regular basis is damaging to the body. This habit is usually accompanied by poor eating habits and depression which lead to a further decline in appearance. Smoking not only causes a decrease of oxygen reaching the skin and other body parts, but also causes wrinkles and a loss of elasticity in the skin.

Personal Hygiene

Keeping your skin, hair and teeth clean and healthy is important in maintaining and prolonging a youthful appearance. Neglect of personal hygiene leads to an unattractive appearance and damage to the body.

Sunlight, Wind and Cold

The sun is thought to be the primary cause of wrinkles, pigment changes and skin cancer. Extended exposure to sun, wind and cold leads to dry skin.

Physical Illness or Disability

Problems with the body's systems or other damage to the body often affect one's appearance e.g. paleness.

Emotional State

How you feel on the inside shows on the outside. Someone who is happy and confident will usually walk tall with a smile and a friendly attitude, whereas someone who is unhappy and depressed will be unmotivated, cranky and may neglect their appearance. Looking good makes you feel good too!

Stress and Fatigue

Stress and fatigue can take their toll on your appearance making you look tense, tired and/or run-down.

WHAT CAN I DO?

The following suggestions may put you on the road to a fresher, younger appearance. You can look better and feel better.

1. Exercise!

Exercise is extremely valuable in forming and maintaining a more youthful appearance. Through regular exercise you may:

- minimize height loss

- improve posture

- increase muscle size

- control fat build-up

- reduce wrinkles

- help prevent age spots

- increase energy

- increase self-esteem

- increase self-confidence

- reduce stress and fatigue

Not only can you look younger through exercise, but you will feel younger too!

2. Eat Well

Your body requires a nutritious diet in order to function properly. Eating well will supply all the nutrients your body needs, avoiding the 'run-down' appearance resulting from an unhealthy diet. (Don't forget to drink plenty of water!) Getting adequate calcium is important and can help prevent height loss and poor posture.

3. Practise Good Hygiene

Keeping clean and taking care of your body greatly enhances your appearance and prevents damage to the body. The main cause of tooth loss is gum (periodontal) disease, which can be prevented through proper hygiene. Use a soft toothbrush, floss daily and use a fluoride toothpaste or mouthwash.

Shampoo regularly to fight dandruff.

Rinse well after washing with soap to prevent drying of the skin.

Treat your skin well — don't use harsh cleansers or products containing alcohol.

4. Protect and Moisturize Skin and Hair

Your hair and skin will benefit from protection, keep them moisturized.

Use a sunscreen [15 SPF (sun protection factor) or more is recommended] when out in the sun to help prevent dryness, wrinkling and age spots.

Use skin lotion as often as needed to moisturize your skin and nails.

Use conditioner on your hair after shampooing to moisturize hair.

Comb hair rather than brush it to discourage breakage.

Limit the use of your hairdryer, and if possible, use at a lower temperature setting to reduce damage to hair.

5. Quit Smoking and Heavy Drinking

Excessive smoking and heavy drinking damage the skin. Quitting now, among other important health benefits, will prevent further damage to the skin.

6. Get Enough Rest and Relaxation

Feeling rested and unstressed prevents a tired, run-down, tense appearance.

7. Update Clothing, Hairstyle, and Make-up

What looked good for you when you were younger probably doesn't suit you now. Experiment to see what suits you best.

Clothing

An updated wardrobe doesn't mean an expensive or flashy one. Choose clothing that suits your figure and proportions — be sure it fits well. If your hair has turned grey, you may want to try something brighter to wear. Look for stylish clothing, but avoid trendy clothes which will be outdated in a year or two.

Hairstyle

A short hairstyle suits many people; it can be flattering and it's easy to take care of. Ask your hairdresser about flattering cuts for older adults. Many new styling products are available such as mousses, gels and sprays — experiment with them.

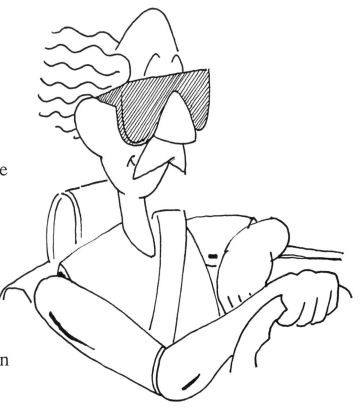

Make-up

Make-up can create a big difference in appearance — experiment! However, for most women, the 'less-is-better' rule applies. Going for a make-over can be a fun way to learn new make-up ideas.

8. Remove Unwanted Hair

There are many methods available, such as bleaching, waxing and electrolysis, to remove or minimize the appearance of unwanted facial hair. Discuss this with your physician.

Most older people are not overly concerned with the age-related changes in their appearance and have a positive view of themselves. However, everyone enjoys looking attractive, healthy and well-groomed. Following the above suggestions can make you look better, feel better, and be a new you!

Did You Know That:

- the average human head contains approximately 75,000 — 120,000 hairs

- a fingernail grows approximately 1/8 of an inch per month or one inch every eight months

- when young, your skin entirely renews itself every 30 days or so; as you age, this renewal process slows down

EATING HABITS

A proper diet is important throughout your lifetime. Seniors, however, need to pay special attention to their food habits since they suffer from malnutrition more than any other age group. This malnutrition is often due to a variety of factors and may go unnoticed and/or untreated for a long period of time. Fortunately, the switch to a healthy diet usually requires just a few changes in your eating habits.

WHAT CHANGES AFFECT MY EATING HABITS AS I AGE?

There are physical changes which occur with aging that affect what you eat and how your body uses your food.

Slower Body Metabolism

A slower *metabolism* means that your body doesn't need as much energy from food to keep your body running smoothly. This results in the need for fewer calories in your diet. Too many calories in your diet will result in a gain in weight. You still need the same amount of *nutrients* however so it is important that you eat the right food.

Loss of Body Tissue

As you age, your body naturally loses tissue. You lose some muscle mass, some bone mass, and your organs become somewhat smaller. This loss of body tissue is normal, very slight, and is no cause for concern. If there are too many calories in your food, this change contributes slightly, along with a slower metabolism, to a weight gain as we age.

Less Efficient Digestive System

Your digestive system doesn't work quite as well as when you were younger. However, for most people there are no large changes in their need for proteins, vitamins and minerals. A healthy diet should provide your body with the nutrients it needs. Chewing and swallowing may become more difficult due to the fact that there is a decrease in the amount of saliva produced by your body. This may have a great effect on your eating habits.

Loss in Senses of Taste and Smell

Older adults often experience a decrease in their ability to taste and smell. This may affect your choice of food and your use of seasonings, such as salt, sugar or gravies.

WHAT ELSE AFFECTS MY EATING HABITS?

There are many factors other than the above age-related changes which may affect the eating habits of the older population.

Loneliness, Depression and Boredom

Older persons living alone often feel that preparing a good meal for one is too much of a bother and find that eating alone is depressing. Depression and boredom tend to reduce one's appetite.

Limited Income

A reduction in income may cause carelessness in shopping for and eating well-balanced meals. With a smaller disposable income it is also possible that the proper storage of food may become a problem, e.g. freezers, refrigerators. Food items may spoil or may have to be purchased in smaller quantities rather than more economical, larger quantities.

Difficulty Getting to Shopping Facilities

Older adults may rely on nearby convenience stores for food, rather than grocery stores, due to a lack of mobility and/or due to transportation problems. Convenience store food is often less nutritious and more expensive than that of grocery stores.

Active/Inactive Lifestyle

Seniors tend to have a less active lifestyle than when they were younger and this will contribute to a weight gain. The amount of food you eat should depend on how active a lifestyle you lead. Exercise is helpful since it improves digestion and relieves constipation, and may reduce depression and increase self-esteem.

Illness, Medication and Physical Disabilities

Illness and some medications may cause nausea, a loss of appetite, and/or poor absorption of nutrients. Because of illness or disability, an individual may depend on others for food choices and/or preparation.

Stress, Sleeping Difficulties and Fatigue

Not enough rest may cause a desire for *stimulants* such as coffee, tea and sweets. Stress, lack of sleep and fatigue may also cause a decrease in appetite or some other change in normal eating habits.

Difficulty Chewing

Healthy food may be replaced with soft, over-processed, often less nutritious food due to missing teeth, sore teeth or gums, or ill-fitting dentures.

Heavy Drinking

Heavy drinking of alcohol is often accompanied by poor eating habits and depression.

Other Factors

Other important factors which affect persons of all age groups and are not especially particular to the older population are:

- food likes/dislikes
- nutrition knowledge
- health beliefs and attitudes
- skill in food preparation
- food advertising

WHAT CAN I DO?

Improving your eating habits is probably not as difficult as you might think.

Canada's Food Guide sets out the guidelines for good nutrition. Following are some suggestions to improve problem areas affecting your eating habits.

1. Eating Well

A variety of food from the four food groups (Canada's Food Guide) will provide your body with the nutrients it requires. Following Canada's Food Guide daily will provide the proper amounts. There are some foods which do not contain very many nutrients and therefore are not included in Canada's Food Guide. These foods are called 'extras' and are often high in fat and sugar. Some examples are candy, pop, alcohol, butter, margarine, and salad dressing.

If you are overweight, following Canada's Food Guide will provide you with adequate nutrients and still allow you to lose weight. If you are not overweight and require additional energy, increase the size and number of servings from each food group and/or add a couple of 'extras'.

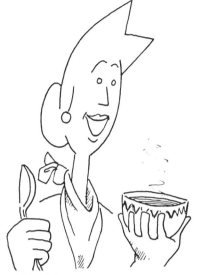

2. Exercise

Exercise and good eating habits compliment each other. Exercise can:

- help in weight control
- increase appetite
- increase energy and self-esteem
- relieve depression and boredom
- improve efficiency of digestive system
- relieve constipation

3. Weight Control

Many older adults have a weight control problem due to a slower *metabolic rate* and reduced physical activity.

Following are some things to keep in mind to ensure that you eat well and avoid unnecessary 'extra' calories:

- follow Canada's Food Guide

- eat less than you used to

- exercise

- avoid the 'extras'

- eat regularly (don't skip meals) — remember, you need fewer calories than when you were younger

- avoid 'crash' and 'fad' diets

- drink at least six glasses of water per day, even if you don't feel thirsty

Tips for Problem Areas

Season foods with herbs, spices, lemon juice, garlic or other items rather than salt, sauces and gravies.

Add fibre in your diet to relieve constipation.

Keep dentures in good condition, and chew food well.

Prepare hard-to-chew foods differently, rather than substitute them with softer, less nutritious foods, i.e. try stewing or roasting meat, then slicing thinly. Graters, blenders and food processors can be handy.

Enjoyable Meals

If living alone, make meal time more enjoyable by making your plate and setting attractive. Sit by your window, watch TV or try taking your lunch to a park. Make eating a social event — invite someone over to share a meal on a regular basis or cook with a group of friends.

Seek Help

See what assistance programmes are available in your area. There are many programmes which provide one or more of the following services:

- inexpensive, nutritious meals

- social interaction with others

- shopping assistance

- counselling

- transportation services

- financial aid

4. See Physician

See your physician about problems affecting your eating habits due to medication and/or illness.

5. Get Enough Rest

Try to get enough rest. If fatigue and/or sleeping problems won't quit, see your physician.

6. Quit Heavy Drinking

If you are a heavy drinker, cut down. Not only is heavy drinking harmful to your body, it often disturbs your eating habits.

Did You Know That:

- it is estimated that humans have the potential to live up to 115, yet life expectancy is now about 74 years

- your body is more than 50 percent water

- experts believe that eating slowly means eating less, (be the first to start eating and the last to finish)

- on the average, a man's blood pressure jumps 6.5 points systolic for every 10 pounds of weight gain

SEXUAL ATTITUDES AND BEHAVIOUR

One of the myths concerning old age in our society is that sexual capabilities, interest and enjoyment are lost with age. The fact is that not only are sexual capabilities and interest present, but sexual activity among older adults should be considered normal and healthy.

WHAT CHANGES AFFECT MY SEXUAL BEHAVIOUR AS I AGE?

Following are some of the physical changes that occur with aging. These changes are normal and need not interfere with sexual activity.

Women May Notice:

- a decrease and/or delay in *vaginal* lubrication

- a decrease in elasticity and ability to expand the vagina

- smaller, less elastic *labia*

- increased time required to reach orgasm

Women may also notice some pain and discomfort in and around the vagina due to physical changes in this area, particularly after menopause. This pain/discomfort can often easily be remedied with the help of your physician.

Men May Notice:

- slower sexual arousal

- increased time required to achieve erection

- full erection often is not attained until just before ejaculation

- erection may be maintained for longer periods of time

- increased time is required following orgasm before erection and ejaculation are again possible

- fewer orgasms

- decreased pleasure with orgasm

The physical changes that occur with age place some restrictions on sexual activities. However, they certainly do not make effective sexual behaviour impossible. In fact, sexual activity can continue long after other functions have begun to decline. An individual is often affected emotionally more than physically by these age-related changes. He/she may feel as if they are losing their sexuality and suffer a decrease in self-esteem. Knowing that these changes are normal and are experienced by others is helpful in letting people become more comfortable with changes in sexual ability.

There may be a slight decline in sexual capabilities with age, however there are many advantages to sex in later life. Older adults are more experienced, are not concerned about pregnancy, and often share a great deal of intimacy. The length of time both partners can stay sexually excited greatly increases, prolonging pleasure for both.

WHAT ELSE AFFECTS MY SEXUAL BEHAVIOUR?

Although sexual capabilities continue into old age, sexual activity tends to diminish. A decrease in sexual activity is much more likely due to a factor or factors other than the physical changes that occur with age, such as the following:

Physical/Mental Illness

Health problems are often present in people over 70 and may prevent effective sexual activity, e.g. arthritis, diabetes.

Social Beliefs and Attitudes

In society, sexual activity in older adults tends to be regarded as improper. The belief that such activity is inappropriate in later years may cause older adults to refrain from sexual activity.

Personal Attitudes

Poor past sexual experiences, religious beliefs and other personal attitudes greatly affect sexual relations in older adults.

Decrease in Marital Satisfaction

It is not uncommon for older couples to experience problems in their marriage, particularly during stressful times such as retirement. A decrease in marital satisfaction often results in reduced sexual activity.

Monotony will often result in less sexual activity, however this boredom has probably been around for a number of years and did not set in with age.

Lack of Partner

The lack or loss of a spouse often causes a great decrease in the sexual activity of an individual.

Poor Self-Image

Changes in physical appearance with age may result in a poor self-image. An individual may feel he/she is no longer attractive to their partner and thus refrains from sexual activity.

Fear of Threat to Health

Sexual activity may be avoided if an individual feels that such activity will endanger their health. e.g. persons with heart trouble or high blood pressure. Sexual activity is usually no more strenuous than climbing a flight or two of stairs, however, if you are concerned, consult your physician.

Lack of Sexual Activity in Previous Years

Patterns of sexual activity throughout life are usually continued into the senior years. Regular sexual activity appears to enhance sexual interest and frequency rather than diminish it.

Fear of Being Unable to Perform

Men may avoid sexual activity if they have recently been unable to perform, rather than risk embarrassment if they encounter the problem again.

Lack of sexual desire could be due to:

- too much caffeine (coffee and tea)
- unbalanced diet
- lack of exercise
- frequent alcohol use
- stress
- fatigue
- some medications

WHAT CAN I DO?

If you are experiencing a lack of desire and/or a lack of sexual activity and it is a problem for you, you may want to look into one or more of the following suggestions:

1. Examine Your Lifestyle

A problem with desire may simply be due to too much coffee or tea, poor eating habits, not enough exercise, alcohol, stress or fatigue.

2. Communicate With Your Partner

Try talking openly with your partner. Withholding your thoughts and feelings can trigger resentment which cools desire.

3. See Your Physician

If you are experiencing problems with desire or performance, your physician may be able to help. Be sure to ask about any medication you are taking that may be affecting you.

4. Counselling

A problem with desire or performance may be psychological. If this seems to be the case, seeing a counsellor may help.

5. Exercise

Studies have shown that people who exercise have more sexual desire than unfit people and that regular exercise can help problems such as impotence, premature ejaculation and the inability to achieve orgasm.

Did You Know That:

- sexual function is one of the last functions to decline with age

- nearly all men experience erection problems at some point in their lives

- the peak age of sexual desire in men is approximately 17 years of age and in women, about 38 years of age

ENERGY

Zip, vigour, pep — these are all terms we use when we talk about how much energy we have. As you age you may find that you do not have the energy for physical activity that you used to. This lack of energy with age is usually not only due to the aging process itself, but due to a combination of factors. Regaining and/or maintaining that youthful zip is possible through the appropriate adjustments of your lifestyle.

WHAT CHANGES AFFECT MY ENERGY AS I AGE?

The amount of energy you have as you age is partially determined by some of the physical changes which occur with age.

Rate of Metabolism

As you age your metabolism naturally slows down, decreasing the amount of oxygen reaching the blood and the amount of carbon dioxide leaving the body. Without as much oxygen and with more carbon dioxide, the body doesn't provide as much energy. This results in a reduction of the amount of energy available for physical activity.

Capacity and Efficiency of Heart and Lungs

Changes in the heart and lungs with age reduce the amount of oxygen and nutrients reaching the body's cells and the amount of waste products leaving the cells. Without as much oxygen or as many nutrients, and with more waste products, the body is unable to function as efficiently. This causes a decline in the amount of energy available for physical activity.

Amount and Strength of Muscle

As you age, you lose muscle mass and muscle strength resulting in less strength and *endurance* during physical activity.

Capacity and Efficiency of Digestive System

The digestive system is one of the systems that becomes less efficient with age. Absorption of nutrients into the blood becomes more difficult, decreasing the quantity of nutrients reaching the body and cells. This results in a decline in the amount of energy available for physical activity.

WHAT ELSE AFFECTS MY ENERGY?

Although you may experience a loss of energy due to the aging process, there are other factors which can affect your energy reserves.

Active/Inactive Lifestyle

The senior years are often accompanied by an inactive lifestyle. Lack of regular exercise speeds up the aging process by further reducing the efficiency of the body's systems. This results in little energy available for physical activity. If an individual is inactive and overweight, he must work even harder to do everyday tasks and has even less energy available for activity. Regular physical activity conditions the body and reduces the amount of energy required to perform tasks and helps the body to develop extra energy.

Eating Habits

Poor eating habits deprive your body of the nutrients it needs in order to sustain healthy functions and supply you with energy. Feeling tired may be due to a lack of nutrients important for energy, such as iron, magnesium or potassium.

Depression and Self-esteem

Depression and low self-esteem often are accompanied by a 'run-down' sensation and a lack of energy.

Stress and Fatigue

Stress and fatigue can deplete your energy supply leaving you constantly listless and tired.

Pain/Illness/Medication

Certain pains, illnesses or medications may cause a lack of energy and/or strength.

Sleeping Difficulties

A lack of sleep drains your body of energy. You need sufficient rest in order to feel energetic.

Digestive Difficulties

Problems with digestion may deprive your body of needed nutrients despite a good diet, resulting in a lack of energy.

Smoking and Drinking Habits

Smoking is harmful to the lungs, reducing the amount of oxygen reaching the blood and thereby decreasing the amount of energy available for activity. Drinking alcohol depresses the amount of sugar in your blood. This sugar is required for energy. Heavy drinking habits are often accompanied by poor eating and sleeping habits, and depression, which all tend to reduce one's energy.

WHAT CAN I DO?

A loss of energy with age can be frustrating for some people as they find they are unable to do some of the things they used to. Don't despair however, if a lack of energy is making you feel 'old'. The following suggestions can be very helpful in regaining and/or maintaining a youthful energy boost for years to come.

1. Exercise

Exercise is extremely valuable in improving one's energy level. Through exercise you may:

- improve respiratory system capacity and efficiency
- improve cardiovascular system capacity and efficiency
- improve digestive system capacity and efficiency
- strengthen muscles
- reduce mental and physical fatigue
- improve self-esteem
- improve sleep

With regular exercise, you may remain spry and energetic almost indefinitely.

2. Eat Well

Perk up your body and your energy with a healthy diet. Eating properly nourishes your body with the nutrients you need to function and feel well.

3. See Your Physician

If certain pains, illnesses and/or medications are affecting your energy reserves, discuss it with your physician.

4. Stay Positive

Keeping a positive attitude is important in remaining energetic throughout life.

5. Keep that Vitality

To avoid depression and increase energy, get mentally and physically active. Develop new interests, get involved in activities and increase social contact to keep that vitality fresh!

6. Get Enough Rest

Adequate rest is necessary in order to feel energetic during the day. If you suffer from sleeping difficulties, see your physician.

7. Quit Smoking and Heavy Drinking

Prevent further damage to your lungs and improve your respiratory system by quitting now. Drinking alcohol in moderation, rather than drinking heavily, will prevent further damage to your body and will likely improve eating and sleeping habits, as well as reduce depression.

You can't turn back the clock, but you can wind it up again!

Did You Know That:
- for most people, their energy peaks at mid-morning and sometime again in late afternoon (schedule activities that require the most energy and attention at these times)

- alcohol depresses your blood sugar or the fuel that your body needs for power. When you drink alcohol, your energy level goes down

- a cool bath (80° - 90°F) acts as a tonic because it stimulates the nerves

REFERENCES

Atchley, R. C. (1987). Aging: Continuity & change (2nd ed.). Belmont, California: Wadsworth.

Boston Women's Health Book Collective. (1984). The new our bodies, ourselves (rev. ed.). New York: Simon & Schuster.

Cape, R. (1978). Aging: Its complex management. Hagerstown, Maryland: Harper & Row.

Holbrook, S., & Merry, G. (1984). Improving with age: How to enjoy your senior years. Toronto: Deneau.

Keough, C. (Ed.). (1987). Future youth: How to reverse the aging process. Emmaus, Pennsylvania: Rodale Press.

McKenzie, S. C. (1980). Aging and old age. Glenview, Illinois: Scott, Foresman and Company.

Spence, A. P. (1989). Biology of human aging. New Jersey: Prentice-Hall.

Spirduso, W. W., & Eckert, H. M. (Eds.). (1989). Physical activity and aging. Champagne, Illinois: Human Kinetics Books.

Subak-Sharpe, G., & Weiss, R. J. (Eds.). (1988). Complete guide for health and well-being after 50. New York: Random House.

The Ontario Milk Marketing Board. (1984). A nutrition education program for health professionals. Mississauga: Author.

Tomb, D. A. (1984). Growing old. New York: Viking Penguin.

Wantz, M. S., & Gay, J. E. (1981). The aging process: A health perspective. Cambridge, Massachusetts: Winthrop.

Whitney, E. N., & Hamilton, E. M. N. (1984). Understanding nutrition (3rd ed.). St. Paul, Minnesota: West.

SECTION 2

PSYCHOLOGICAL CHANGES

ARE THERE PSYCHOLOGICAL CHANGES ASSOCIATED WITH AGING?

YES.

Aging Usually Causes:

- some difficulty in communicating

- some difficulty in learning new information

- some changes in an individual's self-concept

- a change in an individual's social roles and relationships

Aging May Also Bring:

- emotional changes

- changes in self-confidence

In this section we will take a look at each one of these psychological changes which can occur as we grow older.

COMMUNICATION

HOW DOES AGING AFFECT COMMUNICATION?

- some seniors experience hearing difficulties

- some seniors experience speech difficulties

HEARING DEFICITS

- difficulty in hearing is the second most common condition in the elderly (arthritis is first)

- approximately 13 per cent of seniors over 65 show advanced signs of hearing loss

Possible Causes:

- impacted ear wax

- stiffening of the small bones in the ear

- ear infection

- some medications cause problems with hearing (ask your physician about the medication you are taking)

You May Notice:
- difficulty in hearing high-frequency consonants such as s , z , t , f , g

- difficulty in hearing the difference between certain one syllable words such as sit and fit

- women's speech is sometimes harder to understand because of their higher-pitched voices

WHAT CAN I DO?

1. Hearing aids are available and are quite effective.

2. Lip reading can also help in understanding what people are saying.

3. Medical intervention can sometimes help.

When Speaking To Someone With A Hearing Deficit:
- lower the pitch of your voice

- speak louder

- speak slowly

- look directly at the person

SPEECH DEFICITS

Possible Causes
- tooth loss and/or adaptation to dentures

- in some cases, strokes may impair certain areas in the brain which are responsible for speech production and comprehension

WHAT CAN I DO?

1. Speech/language therapy, whereby the person is taught how to adapt to these changes in order to facilitate speech production, is useful.

LEARNING

DO OLDER ADULTS HAVE MORE DIFFICULTY LEARNING NEW INFORMATION?

YES and NO.

Although seniors tend to have more problems than younger people learning new information, the difference is not necessarily due to age itself. The difference is mostly due to the fact that younger people are constantly learning new information either in school or in a work setting. Little or no difference has been found between young and older people's learning ability, if seniors are also learning new information on a regular basis.

What Else Effects My Learning Efficiency?

Practice
The more you practice, the better you become at learning.

Health
Good health increases learning efficiency.

Motivation
You have to want to learn.

Education Level
People with more education sometimes learn more easily.

Intelligence
Intelligence level is important, however it is not the only factor.

Confidence
The more you have to learn something, the easier it will be to learn; the more you learn, the more confidence you will gain.

Learning Styles
The way you go about learning something is also important.

Facts About Learning And Memory:

1. After teaching older adults learning strategies, such as visual techniques, they can learn new information almost as well as younger people.

2. Being out of school for a long time and/or not learning new information on a regular basis affects learning efficiency; daily practise brings improvement.

3. There is very little difference between the short-term memory of older and younger people.

4. Although the short-term memory capacity is practically the same in young and older people, seniors are more easily distracted by thoughts or ideas they may have while doing something.

5. You are not losing your memory; you must simply change or adapt to how you have to retrieve the information.

You May Notice:

- that you may have more difficulty in retrieving information

- that you may be more easily distracted by other thoughts

- that it takes more time to learn new information

WHAT CAN I DO TO SHARPEN UP MY LEARNING AND MEMORY CAPABILITIES?

1. To learn something new, work at your own pace and try to avoid distractions.

2. To remember someone's name, for example, you may try going through the letters of the alphabet one by one in order to remember the first letter of the person's name.

3. To remember the time of your appointment, picture where you were when you wrote the time down in your calender, and picture if it was written in pen or in pencil, etc. These cues may help you retrieve the necessary information.

4. To remember something someone said to you, picture where you were standing, who else was with you, what you answered to the person speaking to you, etc.

5. The more you practise, the easier it will become for you to learn new information and to remember things.

6. Keep healthy and in good physical condition.

SOCIAL ROLES AND RELATIONSHIPS

DO SOCIAL ROLES AND RELATIONSHIPS CHANGE AS PEOPLE AGE?
YES.

The Aging Parent Will Probably:
- become a grandparent

- have an aging spouse

- have suffered the loss of a spouse by divorce or death

- have found a new partner

- see fewer friends

- find the opportunity to develop new friendships

Most Older Adults:
- prefer to live in separate households

- participate actively in the community

- engage in a wide range of social activities

- are not isolated from friends or family

Things To Remember

1. Not all older people want to be grandparents.

2. Some older married couples report a deterioration in their marriage.

3. Almost half of the elderly suffer the death of a spouse.

4. In a couple, the man will usually die before the woman.

5. Widows and widowers often suffer a break-off in friendships they had with other married couples before the death of their spouse.

6. After retirement or widowhood, friendships are extremely important for a person's general well-being.

7. The family is the most frequently used source of social support for older people.

EMOTIONS

ARE THERE COMMON EMOTIONAL REACTIONS IN OLDER ADULTS?

YES.

Common Emotions:

- fear of being abandoned

- fear of loneliness

- anger because of the way older adults are treated

- frustration caused by growing old

- a sense of not wanting to burden other

- regret for past actions or words that were intended but left unsaid

- sadness

- anxiety due to changes in the body, mind, relationships, feelings, and the environment

Important Factors For Well-being:

- good health

- socio-economic status

- degree of social interaction

- marital status

- housing

- availability of transportation

Things To Remember:

1. Older adults experience emotions which are just as strong as emotions in younger people.

2. Since the body takes longer to return to normal in older adults, the duration of the emotional experience seems to be longer, and there is less of a variety of strong emotions within the same day.

3. Identical events cause different emotions over time.

4. Seniors are less likely to describe themselves as 'very happy' but are more likely to report a higher level of overall 'life satisfaction'.

SELF-CONCEPT AND SELF-ESTEEM

Self-concept simply means how you see yourself.

DOES THE SELF-CONCEPT OF AN INDIVIDUAL CHANGE OVER TIME?:

YES and NO.

Yes

Your self-concept will usually include your role in society, which is something that does change.

Biological changes such as loss of strength, stamina, and youthful looks also affect the way you see yourself.

No

The personality traits of your self-concept do not change. For example if you considered yourself to be anxious, curious, hardworking, and gentle when you were younger, you are likely to see yourself this way in your senior years as well.

SELF-ESTEEM

Self-esteem means the basic feeling you have of yourself.

Factors That Predict Self-Esteem:

- education

- type of occupation

- present level of income

- types of leisure activities

- interpersonal success with family and friends

Facts:

1. Self-esteem does not seem to change with age, probably because the elderly choose to look at the positive aspects of growing old.

2. The healthier you are, the less likely you are of having negative self-esteem.

3. A positive attitude toward aging maintains high self-esteem.

REFERENCES

Belsky, J. (1984). The psychology of aging theory, research & practice. Monterey California: Brooks Cole Publishing Co..

Birren, J. E., & Schaie, K. W. (1985). Handbook of the psychology of aging (2nd ed.). New York: Van Nostrand Reinhold Co..

Krauss Whitbourne, S. (1986). Adult development (2nd ed.). New York: Praeger Special Studies.

Maddox, G. L. (1987). The encyclopedia of aging. New York: Springer.

Schulz, R., & Ewen, R. B. (1988). Adult development & aging: Myths and emerging realities. New York: McMillan Publishing Co..

Section 3

QUALITY OF LIFE

STRESS

Stress is the way you react (physically or emotionally) to change, pleasant or unpleasant. Stress can be either positive or negative.

Positive Stress

Stress can help you concentrate, perform, play and work better.

Some people do their best work under pressure.

Negative Stress

Too much stress over a long term, on the other hand, can often cause physical ailments such as tension headaches and heart attacks.

Stress Awareness

The first thing to do is to try to identify the events in your life that cause you to feel stress.

The next thing to do is to try to focus on how your body feels in these situations.

The key to handling stress is learning how to cope with it.

Coping with stress simply means learning to identify the problems and finding solutions. Here are a few hints on how you can reduce the negative effects of stress:

1. Avoid Hassles

If riding the bus during rush-hour 'drives you up the wall' make an effort to travel outside of the peak hours of traffic.

If rushing to get somewhere on time makes you very anxious, try leaving earlier or allowing yourself more time to get there.

2. Control Your Lifestyle Changes

If one aspect of your life changes, do what you can to limit any other changes in your life for a little while.

If you have recently retired or suffered the loss of someone close to you, make an effort to continue the things that bring you pleasure.

3. Take A Break

Sometimes you need a little distance from your problems to work them out correctly.

Take a few minutes by yourself, sit down, relax and figure out what needs to be done now, and what can wait until later on.

Take it one step at a time.

4. Find Help

If you notice that you are unable to cope with your problem by yourself, you may want to consult your doctor in order to eliminate any medical reasons for your problem.

If you don't have a physical problem, you could try talking to someone who can listen to you and understand your feelings. This person could be a good friend, a relative, or a professional counsellor.

Minor Symptoms That May Indicate Signs Of Stress

- rashes
- more colds than normal
- hives
- heart palpitations
- eyelid twitching
- increased sweating
- cold hands or feet
- feeling that things are getting out of control
- muscle aches
- allergies
- jaw pain
- facial tics
- difficulty swallowing
- nausea, vomiting

- cold, clammy hands

- frustration

- anxiety

- irritability

Remember
What may be a symptom of stress in one person could be nothing more than a normal reaction for someone else.

HOW TO COPE

There are many different ways to deal with stress, some of these are good and others are bad. For example:

Bad Ways Of Coping:

- **alcohol:** drinking to feel better

- **tobacco:** smoking to relieve tension

- **medication:** abusing aspirin, sleeping pills, tranquillizers, etc.

- **over-eating and drinking:** using food or coffee, tea, etc., to make yourself feel better

- **fault-finding:** complaining, criticizing

- **passivity:** hoping it gets better without doing anything about it

- **revenge:** getting even, being sarcastic

- **stubbornness:** demanding your way

- **tantrums:** yelling, pouting, swearing

- **worrying:** imagining the worst

- **withdrawal:** avoiding the situation

Good Ways Of Coping:

- **music:** listening to the radio

- **getaways:** seeing a movie

- **learning:** reading, joining a club

- **assertiveness:** saying "no" respectfully

- **expression:** showing and sharing feelings

- **imagination:** looking for the humour in things

- **nourishment:** eating nutritious food

- **relaxation**: taking a warm bath or breathing deeply

- **stretching**: taking short breaks throughout the day in order to stretch your muscles

- **exercise**: regular exercise is a great way to cope with stress (try the exercise programme in this manual)

Stress is a major cause of alcoholism, ulcers, high blood pressure, headaches, heart attacks and suicides. In order to avoid the impact of stress on your mind and body you must learn how and when to relax.

There are many important steps that can help you beat stress, here are just a few that you may want to put into practice:

- exercise
- cut out caffeine
- don't use salt at the table.
- don't skip meals
- learn to relax (see relaxation exercises, Chapter 6)
- develop a sense of humour
- make decisions
- try a massage
- know your own weaknesses
- avoid alcohol
- avoid gossip
- take medication with care
- try yoga
- spoil yourself

REFERENCES

Ballance, S. (1990). Stress Seminar presented at Laurentian University, Sudbury, Ontario, Canada.

Coffey, L. (1982). Be restored to health: How to manage stress, heal yourself and be whole again. New York: Lewis Ballantine Books.

Hanson, P. (1985). The joy of stress. Hanson Stress Management Organization. 5 Thornbury Crescent, Islington Ontario. M9A 2M1

Maddox, G. L. (1987). The encyclopedia of aging. New York: Springer Publishing Co..

Maddox, G. L., & McRae, R. R. (Ed.). (1987). Stress and stressors. The Encyclopedia of Aging. New York: Springer Publishing Co..

CHAPTER 4

DRESSING FOR FITNESS

We all enjoy dressing nicely because when we look good we feel good. If you exercise in an exercise suit that makes you feel good, you feel confident. It is necessary to feel good about yourself, but if you don't dress properly, your body will soon tell you. You could end up with sore feet, stomach cramps, sores or even serious injuries as a result of poorly fitting clothes or shoes. "To look nice is good, but to feel good is great!"

WHERE SHOULD I GO TO PURCHASE EXERCISE CLOTHING?

You can find exercise clothing in most stores almost anywhere, but a specialty shop may often have an experienced staff member who will fit your clothing properly. This person may help you find the most suitable shoes, suit, or accessories for the type of exercise that you choose. Shop around — compare prices of the same brand of clothes in various stores. You need not spend a lot of money in order to get what you want.

WHAT SHOULD I WEAR ON MY FEET?

Since in your lifetime you may walk approximately 120,000 miles, it is reasonable to say that you should take care of your feet. After all, "a pretty face starts with your feet!"

As we age, we sometimes suffer many problems with our feet (e.g. bunions, ingrown toenails) and proper footwear becomes even more important.

Good quality running shoes are your most important purchase for exercise.

Your feet must be comfortable and well supported to enable you to enjoy 'getting in shape'. When shopping for running shoes, you should remember to:

1. Buy shoes with a soft, flexible upper part, a firm but flexible, impact-absorbing sole and a cushioned arch.

2. Buy leather or canvas which enable the shoe to breathe like your skin. Leather shoes are more expensive but will last longer; they will stretch and contract as your feet swell and change while you exercise. With leather shoes you are less likely to have problems with heat and moisture buildup or with bacteria irritating your feet.

3. Make sure your shoes have a well-padded tongue.

4. Buy an all-purpose running shoe rather than one designed specifically for one sport.

5. Avoid toes that are pointed; your foot is squarish in shape so pointed shoes will probably constrict your feet.

6. Arthritic fingers make it difficult to tie laces so you may consider running shoes with Velcro straps.

When you purchase shoes remember these suggestions during your fitting:

1. Buy them in the afternoon when your feet are swollen to their maximum size.

2. Wear the same socks that you will wear to exercise.

3. Your right foot is usually a little larger than your left so determine your largest foot and have the shoe fit to it rather than to the smaller foot.

4. Be sure to try on both shoes and walk around for five or ten minutes. Make sure there are no pressure points. You need to be sure that, as your feet swell from walking, the shoes still fit property.

5. The tip of your toe should not touch the end of the shoe nor should your feet feel cramped.

The shoes should be roomy enough to wiggle your toes. They *must* feel good — you will wear them often as you exercise.

6. Be sure to lace the shoe while sitting, keeping your feet flat on the floor. Place your heel so that your foot is firmly back in the shoe and lace it snugly. Crossing your legs while tying your shoes is not a good practice.

If, after you have worn your shoes for a length of time, you notice the heels wearing on one side, it is advisable to have them repaired or replaced so you do not risk injury. A shoe that does not lie flat on the floor will hinder the proper alignment of ankles, knees and hips.

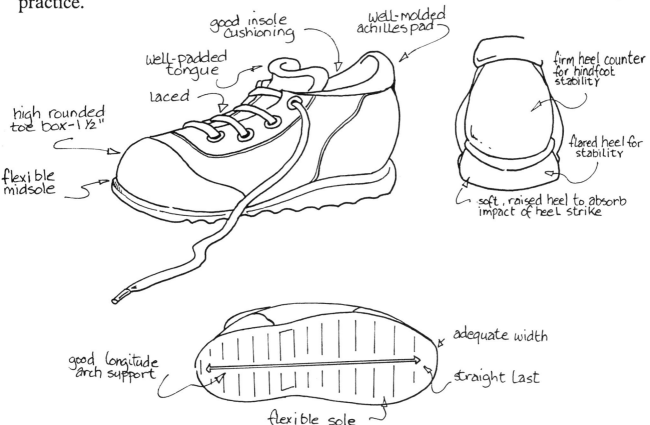

WHAT OTHER CLOTHING IS RECOMMENDED?

There is an extensive variety of exercise clothing in the stores. It is important to wear the appropriate clothing but remember that nice-looking clothes will often help you feel better as well.

Socks

Socks should always be clean and soft, made of cotton or wool rather than nylon which traps heat and moisture causing irritation or itching. Holes in your socks will likely make your feet uncomfortable just as a lump from a darned sock will hurt sometimes. Loose socks which don't constrict the feet or ankles will help your feet feel good. Remember never to use a garter or an elastic to hold up droopy socks. Stockings or pantihose will make you hot and uncomfortable while exercising.

Outerclothing

A loose-fitting sweat-suit or jogging suit is appealing and functional. Again, cotton or wool are fabrics which breathe and allow heat and moisture to escape. These fabrics are a little more expensive but will last a

long time. Nylon does not breathe as well and may result in excess perspiration. Remember, you will be exercising and wool will be warm — perhaps too warm for this purpose. Some tops are zippered only part way down and are then pulled on or off over the head. These look nice but are sometimes very difficult to get on or off.

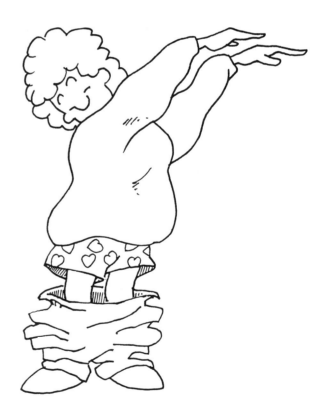

The bottoms or pants don't have to match the top but must be comfortable. Pants usually have an elastic waistband and it is critical that this band be snug so the pants don't fall down. Make certain that this elastic is not so tight as to be uncomfortable. The most important part of the pants is the waistband, so choose it carefully! Sometimes these

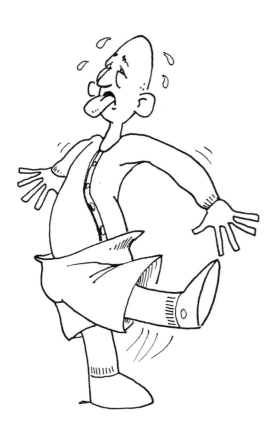

suits are a little too long in the legs but they can easily be shortened. Remember, comfort is the key but your exercise clothing should be moderately priced, washable and suited to you.

Underclothes

You will be involved in rigorous physical activity so if you are a woman, you may want an exercise bra with extra support. Brassieres with underwires are not recommended. Men also may find that an athletic supporter will make them more comfortable during the exercise class. Make sure you do not wear long underwear when exercising — put it on when you have finished, it will help to allow your body to cool down slowly. Your choice of underwear should include articles which are made of cotton rather than synthetic materials so that your body heat and moisture are able to escape.

Your exercise class will be more enjoyable if you take some time to dress properly and take care of yourself. Ladies with long hair may wish to tie it back or put it in a ponytail. Those beautiful diamond rings which could scratch or cut someone are best left at home with other constricting jewellery such as bracelets, watches and necklaces. Earrings should be removed — they could easily catch on something as you 'go through your paces'.

If you follow the suggestions that have been discussed, you are well on your way to comfortable, enjoyable and safe exercising. The rest is up to you!

CHAPTER 5

EXERCISING SAFELY

PLEASE READ THIS SECTION CAREFULLY BEFORE STARTING YOUR EXERCISE PROGRAMME.

There is a great deal of scientific evidence that proper exercise produces a positive effect on the body. For them to be effective, exercises should gradually increase in number of repetitions, length of time and tempo. The benefits of exercise will be greater if they are similar to the regular movements required for your daily activities.

Your body is made for movement. It can become 'out of tune' and cause problems if you do not exercise regularly. If your body is 'out of tune' and you suddenly perform a physical activity which you are not used to, you place your body at risk for pain or even injury. The severity of the pain or injury will depend on your level of 'unfitness' and the manner in which the exercises were performed.

Nevertheless, there are some exercises or movements which can be risky for most people.

The following exercises or movements are considered high risk and should be avoided.

MOVEMENTS THAT MAY BE HARMFUL	WHY THIS MOVEMENT MAY BE HARMFUL	OTHER EXAMPLES OF THIS TYPE OF MOVEMENT
Deep Knee Bends 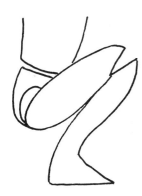	- may place excessive strain on the knee - may cause the knee to become unstable - may damage cartilage of the knee	- duck walk - squatting - kneeling and bending backward
Toe Touches with Straight Legs and Knees Locked 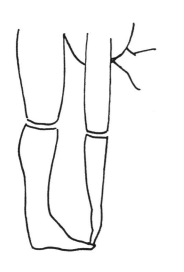	- may cause injury to lower back - may overstretch lower back muscles - hyperextends the knee joint	- sitting on the floor leaning forward to touch toes with legs straight

MOVEMENTS THAT MAY BE HARMFUL	WHY THIS MOVEMENT MAY BE HARMFUL	OTHER EXAMPLES OF THIS TYPE OF MOVEMENT
Backward Head Bends 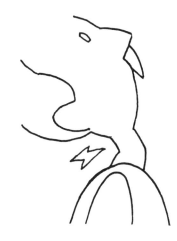	- when excessive, may lead to displaced or damaged vertebrae and discs - may lead to pressure on a nerve (*pinched nerve*)	- back bends - full neck circles with backward head bend - backward rotation of the upper body
Fast, Sharp or 'Bouncing' Movements 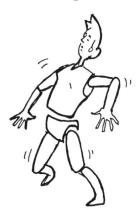	- may cause strain and injury to cartilage, muscles, ligaments and tendons - may cause loss of balance	- short, sharp 'punching' movements - jerky trunk twisting - 'bouncing' while stretching

MOVEMENTS THAT MAY BE HARMFUL	WHY THIS MOVEMENT MAY BE HARMFUL	OTHER EXAMPLES OF THIS TYPE OF MOVEMENT
Any Stretching or Balancing Movement Involving 2 People 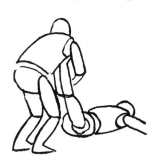	- may cause injury to your partner (one is often unaware of the physical capacity of partner)	- split-leg rowing - both partners supporting each other while balancing - one partner pushing or pulling the other while stretching
Exaggerated Front Lunges 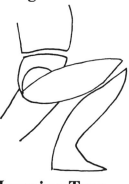	- may cause too much strain on the knee joint (knee should only slightly pass beyond your toes)	- exaggerated side lunges
Jumping-Type Activities (High Impact)	- may cause strain and injury to cartilage, ligaments and tendons - may damage bone	

MOVEMENTS THAT MAY BE HARMFUL	WHY THIS MOVEMENT MAY BE HARMFUL	OTHER EXAMPLES OF THIS TYPE OF MOVEMENT
Sit Ups, Legs Straight 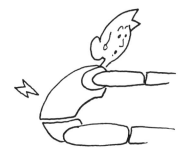	- may cause the lower back to arch - may cause excessive strain on the ligaments, tendons, muscles and discs - may lead to lower back pain and problems	- straight leg lifts, lying on your back
Holding Breath During Exercise (Valsalva Manoeuvre) 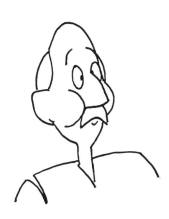	- slows down the blood returning to the heart - increases blood pressure - may cause damage to the blood vessels - may cause dizziness or fainting	- some isometric exercises - explosive type of movement during activity

MOVEMENTS THAT MAY BE HARMFUL	WHY THIS MOVEMENT MAY BE HARMFUL	OTHER EXAMPLES OF THIS TYPE OF MOVEMENT
Lowering Trunk and Head Below Waist Level 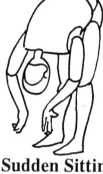	- may cause dizziness and fainting	
Sudden Sitting or Standing Still Immediately Following Strenuous Exercise	- may cause blood to pool in the extremities - may cause dizziness and fainting	

It should be noted that there are four regions of the body which are particularly vulnerable to injury from sudden unaccustomed movement. Therefore caution should be used when doing any exercise for these parts for the first 3 or 4 weeks of a fitness programme. These four regions are:

1. Neck

2. Shoulder

3. Lower Back

4. Knees

Consequently, strength and flexibility exercises for these regions should be done slowly and gradually and performed according to the specific instructions in this manual.

Exercise can also be harmful in the manner in which it is done. If a specific exercise or movement is performed too rapidly, with a large number of repetitions, for a long period of time, without adequate recovery time, a painful injury can occur. This is called the over-use syndrome. Some of the more common types of injury are shin splints, tennis elbow, golf elbow and hair-line fractures.

To avoid an over-use injury, remember that the older you get, the longer it takes to recover from an exercise session. The longer and more strenuous the work-out, the longer the recovery period. When starting a fitness programme, there is risk in doing any exercise if the following rules are not followed:

1. Always increase the repetitions very gradually over the first 4 or 5 weeks.

2. Increase the tempo only after doing the exercise for 4 or 5 weeks.

3. Depending on the exercise, limit the number of repetitions (4) when doing exercises to which you are not accustomed.

The most common danger is rushing into a fitness programme and pushing yourself too hard to achieve a high level of fitness. In the long run, the risk of pain or injury is not worth it. **It is not true that for an exercise to be beneficial it has to hurt.** On the contrary, you advance faster and further by taking it slowly and easily at the beginning.

Finally, in order to eliminate most of the risk it is essential that you consult with your physician before starting any fitness programme. Make sure that you inform your physician of any and every past injury, illness or organic disorder, no matter how unimportant it seems.

The programme designed in this manual provides you with the least risk. None of these exercises, if performed according to the specific instructions, should offer any risk to any independently active person who has received their physician's approval.

More Points to Remember:

DO NOT:

- start an exercise programme without consulting your physician

- exercise without an adequate warm up

- exercise without an adequate cool down

- exercise immediately following a meal

- exercise on the floor without a mat

- use unstable equipment, e.g. a chair without rubber feet

- exercise irregularly (you should exercise 3 to 4 times per week)

- compete with others — DO COMPETE WITH YOURSELF

- follow exercise programmes in magazines or books without consulting your physician

- do any movements described above

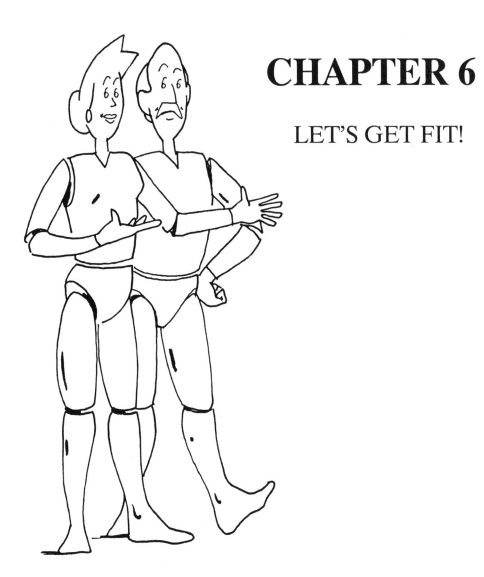

CHAPTER 6

LET'S GET FIT!

Section 1

GOOD BREATHING TECHNIQUES

Good breathing habits play a very important role in your daily routine. Unfortunately breathing habits are neglected by most people.

As you age your breathing becomes more shallow and your body uses the air you breathe less efficiently. It is therefore important to develop good breathing habits as you grow older.

You are encouraged to practise and use proper breathing habits on an everyday basis whether you are active or resting. Try this 'deep breathing' exercise and notice how relaxed it makes you feel.

When you first practise 'deep breathing' make sure that you are either sitting or lying down. If your body is not used to taking in so much oxygen, *hyperventilation* could occur.

- gently place both hands on your stomach

- slowly breathe in through your nose making sure that you expand both your chest and your stomach (you will feel your hands go up); breathe out through your mouth, making sure that you completely empty your chest and stomach (this time you should feel your hands go down)

- breathing out should take about three times as long as breathing in

At first you may find it difficult to use this 'deep breathing' on a regular basis. However, if you practise it several times a day, it will become more natural for you and you will eventually breathe this way without having to think about it.

While following the exercise programme in this book, keep the following points in mind:

1. There are exercises in this chapter which include instructions on when and how to breathe. This allows for safer and more beneficial results. Please follow these instructions closely.

2. The other exercises give you no instructions on breathing. Your body will naturally choose the proper breathing pattern. Have confidence in your body's decision!

3. While exercising you should never hold your breath. This results in an increase in blood pressure which may lead to discomfort or even more dangerous consequences.

4. Do not perform any exercise which interferes with good breathing for a long period of time.

5. Do not wear tight-fitting clothes which may interfere with your breathing, e.g. tight-fitting belts and tight-fitting bras.

6. It is important to exercise in a room with good air circulation allowing for proper air exchange.

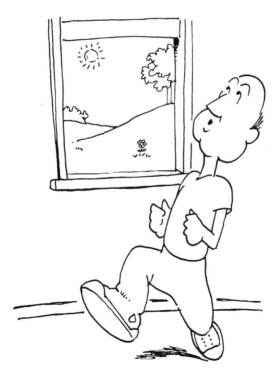

Section 2

UNDERSTANDING THE EXERCISE PROGRAMME

WHY SHOULD I EXERCISE?

Although aging is accompanied by a gradual loss of physical capacity, it is encouraging to know that regular exercise can help you improve or maintain your physical well-being. It also has the added benefit of contributing to your mental and spiritual health.

This chapter focuses on making you aware of the different aspects of fitness. It presents an exercise programme aimed at helping you get involved and improving your level of fitness. With improved fitness, you will enjoy day-to-day living more and build up enough energy to indulge in other enjoyable activities (sports, walking, gardening, social events, leisure). Fitness also has the added benefit of improving the quality of your relaxation and sleep.

The exercises in this chapter are set up so that each class uses a variety of exercises in a specific order. These exercises are aimed at improving the fitness level of all the systems in the body (heart, lungs, muscles, etc.) at the same time allowing exercising to be safe and enjoyable. It is important that you closely follow the instructions as well as the order of the exercises as they are presented in this chapter.

WHAT SHOULD I KNOW ABOUT THIS EXERCISE PROGRAMME?

The programme in this chapter includes three important parts. Each of these parts contains two headings which focus on exercising different systems in your body.

In this book the term exercise class is often used and refers to one exercise workout, whether it be as a group exercising with a fitness instructor or a person exercising alone.

WARM-UP prepares your body for the *exercise class*.

"LET'S BEGIN" prepares your breathing, blood flow and muscles for exercise.

"LET'S LOOSEN UP" loosens your various joints allowing for freer movement during exercise.

BODY OF THE CLASS is the most important part of the exercise class. It improves the fitness of all the systems in your body (heart, lungs and muscles).

"LET'S ENERGIZE" exercises your heart and lungs.

"LET'S TONE UP" exercises and strengthens your muscles.

COOL-DOWN allows your body to recover slowly from exercise.

"LET'S STRETCH" improves your flexibility (warm muscles stretch more easily than cool muscles) and helps decrease muscle soreness after exercising.

"LET'S RELAX" helps your body systems return to rest, and allows your body and mind to relax (the body and mind are able to relax more easily after exercising).

(For more information on the different aspects of fitness, see Chapter 8).

HOW DO I USE THIS EXERCISE PROGRAMME?

The exercise programme in this chapter is broken down into three levels of difficulty. LEVEL 1 is the easiest, whereas LEVEL 3 is the most difficult. In each level there are five exercise classes (sessions). One session consists of 3 exercise classes per week (preferably on alternate days) and lasts for 4 weeks. The difficulty of the exercise classes also increases from Session 1 to Session 5.

The programme is designed to have you progress through the 5 sessions or a 20-week period. Once you have finished session 1 you will move on to session 2 and so on.

Before starting this or any exercise programme you should consult your physician or a fitness specialist to advise you at what level (1, 2 or 3) you should begin exercising. It is recommended that you start exercising at the beginning of Session 1, Level 1.

As you are going through the exercise programme it is very important that you use a BODY CHECK method to see if you are exercising too hard. These BODY CHECKS should be included in every exercise class in order to decrease the possibility of discomfort, injury or even more dangerous consequences. There are 3 important and easy-to-do body checks that you should learn and understand.

Body Check - Monitor Heart Rate

The heart rate check should be done immediately following the "LET'S ENERGIZE" part of each exercise class. This body check allows you to know how fast your heart is beating. A heart that is beating too quickly is a good indication that you are exercising too hard.

Here are 2 easy ways of measuring your heart rate. You can use the method you prefer.

Method #1:

- place the index and middle finger of your right hand on the Adam's apple of your neck

- move both fingers about 2 inches to the left side of your Adam's apple

- slide both fingers about 1 inch towards your jaw

- your fingers should be placed on the artery of your neck as illustrated in FIGURE 1

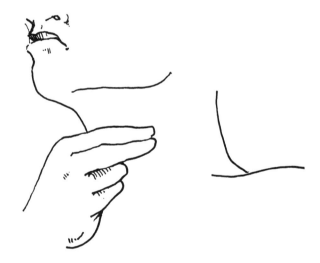

FIGURE 1

- do not apply too much pressure with your fingers since this prevents blood flow in the artery

- with your fingers you should be able to feel a throbbing pulse; this pulse corresponds to the beat of your heart

- counting the first beat as 0, count the number of beats in a period of 10 seconds

- multiply this number by 6 and the answer will give you your heart rate in beats per minute

Method #2:

- place the back of your left wrist in the palm of your right hand as illustrated in FIGURE 2

- bend your right fingers around your left wrist as illustrated in FIGURE 3

- do not apply too much pressure with your fingers since this prevents blood flow in the artery

- using your right index and middle fingers, you should be able to feel a throbbing pulse on the artery of your left wrist; this pulse corresponds to the beat of your heart

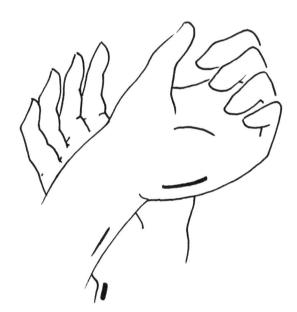

FIGURE 2

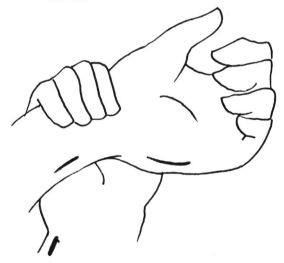

FIGURE 3

- counting the first beat as 0, count the number of beats in a period of 10 seconds

- multiply this number by 6 and this will give you your heart rate in beats per minute

REMEMBER: You should never use your thumb to check your pulse. Your thumb has a pulse itself which may interfere with the correct measurement.

Once you have counted your heart rate, take a look at the following chart.

HEART RATE TARGET ZONE*

AGE (YEARS)	HEART RATE TARGET ZONE (BEATS PER MINUTE)
20-30	138-168
30-40	132-162
40-50	120-150
50-60	108-138
60-70	102-132
OVER 70	102-132

This chart allows you to know approximately what your heart rate should be following the "LET'S ENERGIZE" part of the exercise class.

*Adapted with permission from the HEART RATE TARGET ZONE CHART, Fitness Canada, Fitness & Amateur Sport, Ottawa.

Find where you belong in the age ranges presented in the left column. Look at the corresponding range of values in the right column. This range of values is the recommended heart rate that you should have when you are doing the "LET'S ENERGIZE" part of the exercise class.

Compare your heart rate with the recommended heart rate from the chart. If your heart rate is higher than the recommended heart rate, you are exercising too hard. Be sure to slow down your tempo for the "LET'S ENERGIZE" part of your next exercise class. If your heart rate is lower than the recommended heart rate, you can perhaps speed up your tempo for that part of your next exercise class.

CAREFUL: If you are taking medication (e.g. Inderal) or have any disorder which may affect your heart rate, you should consult your physician for advice on your appropriate heart rate when exercising.

Body Check: Sing

This body check should be done during the "LET'S ENERGIZE" part of the exercise class as indicated in the exercise instructions. This body check allows you to become aware of how fast you are breathing. If you are breathing too quickly it is a good indication that you are exercising too hard.

Here is an easy way of doing this check:

- choose any song

- try to sing the words of this song

- if you become so breathless that you can only sing one-syllable words, then you are exercising too hard

- if this is so, slow down your tempo immediately and continue exercising at a slower pace

Body Check: Overload

Within two days of the exercise class you should do this body check. This body check allows you to know whether your muscles are exercising too hard.

Here is an easy way of doing this body check:

- if you feel too much muscle soreness, muscle pain or stiffness at any of the joints in your body, you are exercising too hard: be sure to lower your number of repetitions and slow down your tempo when you do the "LET'S TONE UP" part of your next exercise class

Before you begin the exercise programme, you should know the meaning of a few terms that you will come across as you go through the instructions.

You will see the term SET appear at the top of some of the exercises. The number of sets refers to the number of times you should do that exercise (including repetitions). When you are instructed to do a number of sets, be sure to rest 5 to 10 seconds between each set. When the number of sets is not indicated, it is always assumed to be 1.

For some of the exercises you will be instructed to use weights. The weights that you are required to use can easily be made using nylons and dried beans or dried soup mix. Place a bag of dried beans into a nylon and tie a knot at both ends (see diagram 5). The amount of weight (beans or dried soup mix) that you put into the stockings will depend on the level at which you are exercising. If you are at LEVEL 2, make the weights using a .9 pound (400 gram) bag of beans in each stocking. If you are at LEVEL 3, make the weights using 2 bags (total weight 1.8 pounds or 800 grams) of beans in each stocking. When you are exercising with weights make sure that you avoid quick, sharp movements. These quick movements can result in injuries to the muscles or the joints. If you have osteoporosis you should consult your physician for specific advice on how to exercise using weights.

For all exercises described in the programme, you should begin by assuming the **BASIC POSITION** unless it is instructed otherwise.

BASIC POSITION

Stand up straight looking straight ahead, with your feet shoulder- width apart, knees slightly bent, and arms hanging loosely alongside your body (as in FIGURE 4).

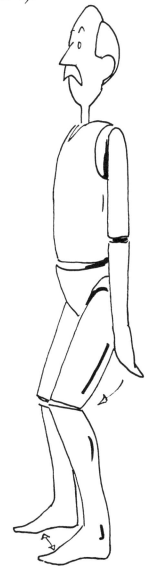

FIGURE 4

LET'S GET FIT - SESSION 1

WARM-UP: LET'S BEGIN!

SESSION 1 - LEVEL I

TOTAL TIME: 4 minutes

PUT ON SOME LIVELY MUSIC.

SIT ON A CHAIR, FEET FLAT ON THE FLOOR. MAKE SURE THAT YOUR BACK AND BOTTOM ARE TOUCHING THE BACK OF THE CHAIR.

1. Step from side to side at a slow, relaxed pace for 30 seconds.

2. Continue to step from side to side and do the following movements for 30 seconds each:

   a) turn head to the right, then to the left

   b) shrug shoulders forward, backward, up and down

   c) swing arms from side to side

   d) kick to the side

   e) with arms alongside body, shake hands

   f) flap your arms as if to fly

   g) gradually, step more slowly

3. Stretch both arms above your head and breathe in deeply (2 times).

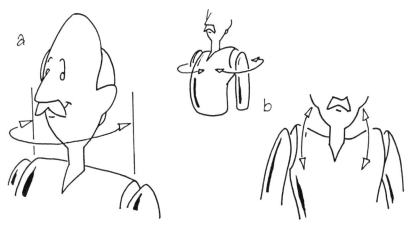
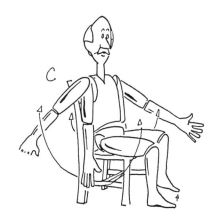

LEVEL II

Do Level I STANDING UP.

LEVEL III

Do Level I STANDING UP.

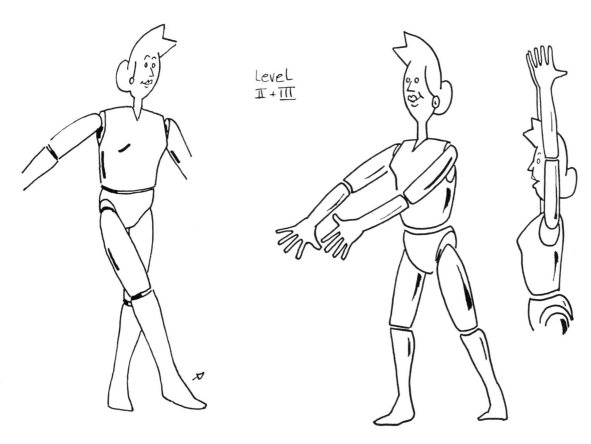

Level
II + III

WARM-UP: LET'S LOOSEN UP!

SESSION 1 - LEVEL I
NECK TURNS:

1. Turn head slowly toward right shoulder.

2. Turn head back to centre.

3. Repeat to other side.

4. Do this sequence 4 times.

LEVEL II
NECK TURNS:

1. Turn head slowly toward right shoulder, trying to look behind you.

2. Turn head back to centre.

3. Repeat to other side.

4. Do this sequence 4 times.

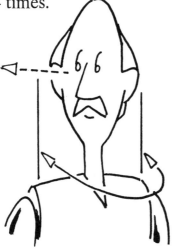

LEVEL III
NECK TURNS:

1. Turn head slowly toward right shoulder, trying to look behind you.

2. Turn head back to centre.

3. Repeat to other side.

4. Do this sequence 6 times.

Remember:
- do not arch back
- keep shoulders still
- do not force this movement

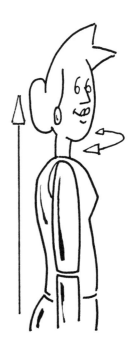

WARM-UP: LET'S LOOSEN UP!

SESSION 1 - LEVEL I
TONGUE EXTENSIONS:

1. Stick your tongue out as far as you can, opening your mouth wide and pulling your chin downward.

2. Relax.

3. Do this sequence 4 times.

LEVEL II
TONGUE EXTENSIONS:

1. Stick your tongue out as far as you can, opening your mouth wide and pulling your chin downward.

2. Relax.

3. Pull closed mouth over to right side as far as possible.

4. Pull closed mouth over to left side as far as possible.

5. Relax.

6. Do this sequence 4 times.

LEVEL III
TONGUE EXTENSIONS:

1. Stick your tongue out as far as you can, opening your mouth wide and pulling your chin downward.

2. Relax.

3. Pull closed mouth over to right side as far as possible.

4. Pull closed mouth over to left side as far as possible.

5. Relax.

6. Do this sequence 6 times.

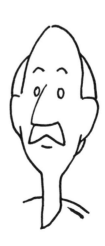
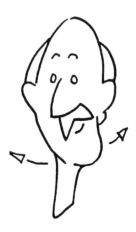

WARM-UP: LET'S LOOSEN UP!

SESSION 1 - LEVEL I
SHOULDER CHA-CHA:

1. Slowly raise (shrug) shoulders toward your ears.

2. Lower your shoulders as far as possible.

3. Return to **BASIC POSITION.**

4. Slowly move both shoulders forward as far as possible.

5. Slowly move both shoulders as far back as possible.

6. Return to **BASIC POSITION.**

7. Do this sequence 4 times.

LEVEL II
SHOULDER CHA-CHA:

1. Place hands on shoulders, keeping elbows up. Keeping hands on shoulders...

2. Slowly raise (shrug) shoulders toward your ears, lifting elbows up.

3. Lower your shoulders as far as possible, pressing elbows down.

4. Slowly bring elbows together in front of you.

5. Slowly bring elbows as far back as possible.

6. Return to starting position.

7. Do this sequence 4 times.

Level I

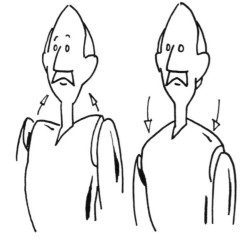
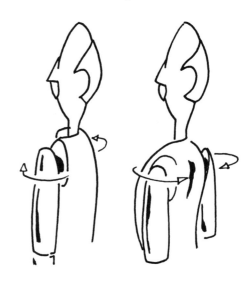

LEVEL III
SHOULDER CHA-CHA:

1. Place hands on shoulders, keeping elbows up. Keeping hands on shoulders...

2. Slowly raise (shrug) shoulders toward your ears, lifting elbows up.

3. Lower your shoulders as far as possible, pressing elbows down.

4. Slowly bring elbows together in front of you.

5. Slowly bring elbows as far back as possible.

6. Return to starting position.

7. Do this sequence 6 times.

Remember:

- keep your neck stretched while you do this exercise

- do not arch back, especially when bringing elbows to the back

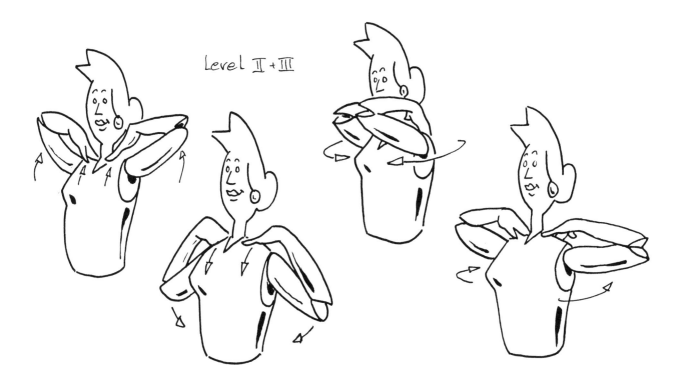

Level II + III

WARM-UP: LET'S LOOSEN UP!

SESSION 1 - LEVEL I
ROCKING HANDS:

1. Clasp hands in front of body, elbows down.

2. Keeping hands clasped, rock hands to right side.

3. Rock hands to left side.

4. Rock hands toward body.

5. Rock hands away from body.

6. Do this sequence 4 times.

LEVEL II
ROCKING HANDS:

1. Place palm against palm in front of body, fingers extended and pointing up, elbows down.

2. Keeping palms and fingers together, bend wrists so that fingers point toward the right elbow.

3. Bend wrist so that fingers point toward left elbow.

4. Bend wrist so that fingers point toward then away from body.

5. Place back of hands together, fingers extended and pointing down.

6. Return to starting position.

7. Do this sequence 4 times.

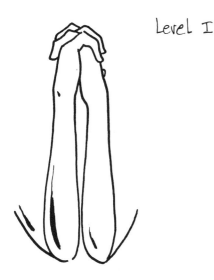

Level I

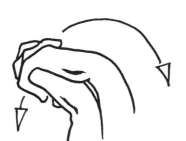

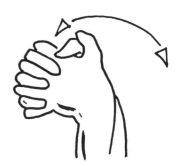

LEVEL III
ROCKING HANDS:

1. Place palm against palm in front of body, fingers extended and pointing up, elbows down.

2. Keeping palms and fingers together, bend wrists so that fingers point toward the right elbow.

3. Bend wrist so that fingers point toward left elbow.

4. Bend wrist so that fingers point toward then away from body.

5. Place back of hands together, fingers extended and pointing down.

6. Return to starting position.

7. Do this sequence 6 times.

Remember:

- try to keep forearms still

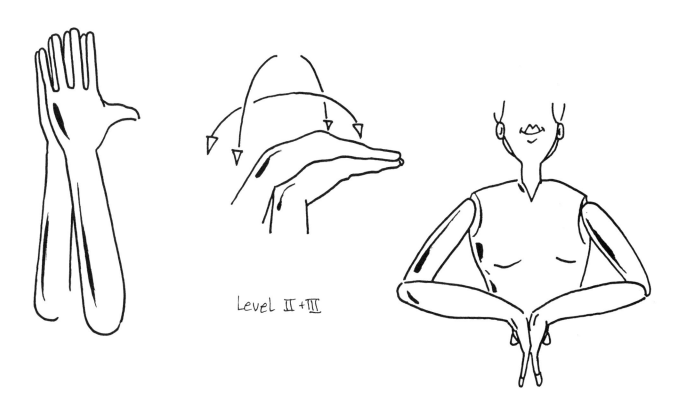

Level II + III

WARM-UP: LET'S LOOSEN UP!

SESSION 1 - LEVEL I
FINGER TO THUMB:

1. Spread the fingers of both hands as far apart as possible.

2. One by one, touch each finger to the tip of your thumb without bending your fingers.

3. Do this sequence 4 times.

LEVEL II
FINGER TO THUMB:

1. Spread the fingers of both hands as far apart as possible.

2. Bend both thumbs to place them on the palms of your hands.

3. One by one, touch each finger to the back of your thumb.

4. Do this sequence 4 times.

LEVEL III
FINGER TO THUMB:

1. Spread the fingers of both hands as far apart as possible.

2. Bend both thumbs to place them on the palms of your hands.

3. One by one, touch each finger to the back of your thumb.

4. Do this sequence 6 times.

Remember:

- keep wrists still
- keep movements slow and smooth
- do not force this movement

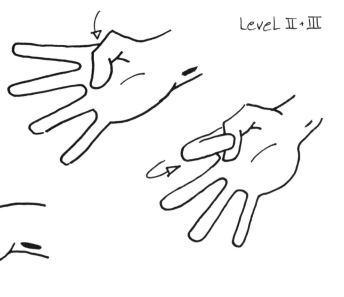

Level I

Level II + III

WARM-UP: LET'S LOOSEN UP!

SESSION 1 - LEVEL I
WAIST TURNS:

1. Place hands on shoulders, keeping elbows to the side and at shoulder level.

2. Keeping hips facing forward, slowly rotate trunk to the right side.

3. Return to starting position.

4. Repeat exercise to the left side.

5. Do this sequence 4 times.

LEVEL II
WAIST TURNS:

1. Stand approximately 1 foot away from the wall, back toward the wall, arms out to sides at shoulder level.

2. Slowly turn upper body to the right to look at the wall, placing both hands on wall.

3. Return to starting position.

4. Repeat exercise to the other side.

5. Do this sequence 4 times.

LEVEL III
WAIST TURNS:

1. Stand approximately 1 foot away from the wall, back toward the wall, arms out to sides at shoulder level.

2. Slowly turn upper body to the right to look at the wall, placing both hands on wall.

3. Return to starting position.

4. Repeat exercise to the other side.

5. Do this sequence 6 times.

Remember:
- do not arch back
- do not force this movement

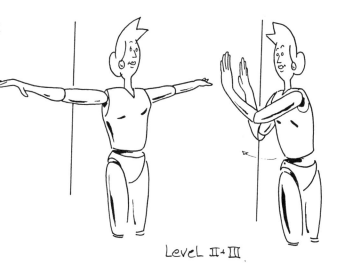

Level II + III

WARM-UP: LET'S LOOSEN UP!

SESSION 1 - LEVEL I
POINT AND STRETCH:

1. Stand with left side toward the wall at arm's length. Place palm flat against the wall at shoulder height.

2. Stretch right leg forward with toes pointed, keeping toes on the floor.

3. Return to starting position.

4. Stretch right leg to the side with toes pointed, keeping toes on the floor.

5. Return to starting position.

6. Stretch right leg to the back with toes pointed, keeping toes on the floor.

7. Return to starting position.

8. Do this sequence 4 times.

9. Turn around, place opposite hand on wall.

10. Repeat exercise with left leg

LEVEL II
POINT AND STRETCH:

1. Stand with left side toward the wall at arm's length. Place palm flat against the wall at shoulder height.

2. Stretch right leg forward with toes pointing forward.

3. Slowly lift leg to knee height.

4. Return to starting position.

5. Repeat this sequence, pointing and lifting leg to the side and to the back.

6. Do this sequence 4 times.

7. Turn around, place opposite hand on wall.

8. Repeat exercise with left leg.

LEVEL III
POINT AND STRETCH:

1. Stand with left side toward the wall at arm's length. Place palm flat against the wall at shoulder height.

2. Stretch right leg forward with toes pointing forward.

3. Slowly lift leg to knee height.

4. Return to starting position.

5. Repeat this sequence, pointing and lifting leg to the side and to the back.

6. Do this sequence 6 times.

7. Turn around, place opposite hand on wall.

8. Repeat exercise with left leg.

Remember:

- do not put weight on pointing foot

- stand up straight

- do not arch back, especially when pointing to the back

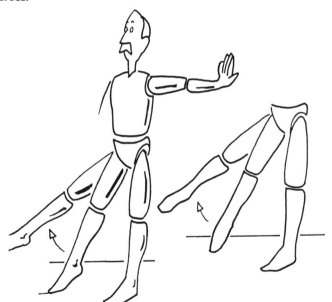
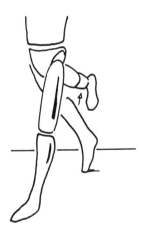

WARM-UP: LET'S LOOSEN UP!

SESSION 1 - LEVEL I
HEEL TOE TOUCH:

1. Stand with left side toward the wall at arm's length. Place palm flat against the wall at shoulder height.

2. Point right foot to the side and touch heel, then toe to floor.

3. Do this sequence 4 times.

4. Return to starting position.

5. Turn around, place opposite hand on wall.

6. Repeat exercise with left leg.

LEVEL II
HEEL TOE TOUCH:

1. Stand facing the wall at arm's length, palms flat against the wall.

2. Bend knees so that knees are just over your toes .

3. Keeping knees bent, go up on the balls of your feet.

4. Place heels on floor.

5. Go back on your heels, lifting toes off the floor.

6. Return to starting position.

7. Do this sequence 4 times.

Level I

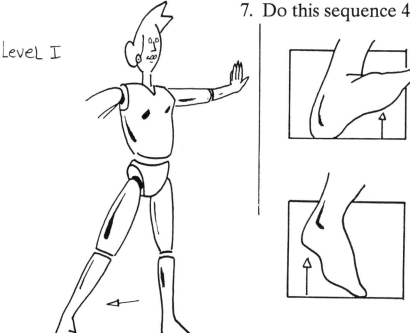

LEVEL III
HEEL TOE TOUCH:

1. Stand facing the wall at arm's length, palms flat against the wall.

2. Bend knees so that knees are just over your toes.

3. Keeping knees bent, go up on the balls of your feet.

4. Place heels on floor.

5. Go back on your heels, lifting toes off the floor.

6. Return to starting position.

7. Do this sequence 6 times.

Remember:

- do not put weight on pointing foot in Level I

- stand up straight

- keep this movement slow and smooth

Level II + III

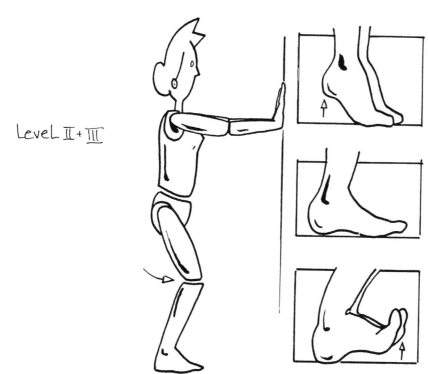

BODY OF THE CLASS: LET'S ENERGIZE!

SESSION 1 - LEVEL I

TOTAL TIME: 5 minutes

PUT ON SOME UPBEAT MUSIC.

SIT ON A CHAIR, FEET FLAT ON THE FLOOR. MAKE SURE THAT YOUR BACK AND BOTTOM ARE TOUCHING THE BACK OF THE CHAIR.

While sitting on a chair, do the following movements for 30 seconds each:

1. Walk on the spot.

2. March, lifting knees and swinging arms.

3. Step side to side, clap hands.

4. Continue stepping side to side, swing arms from right to left at shoulder level.

5. Lifting knees, touch opposite elbow to knee.

6. Walk.

BODY CHECK - SING!

7. Lift right knee, clap hands under thigh. Repeat with left leg.

8. Continue lifting knees, touch opposite hand to foot swinging arms from side to side.

9. Walk slowly.

10. Tap toes.

Stretch both arms above your head and breathe in deeply (2 times).

BODY CHECK - MONITOR HEART RATE!

LEVEL II

TOTAL TIME: 6 minutes

Do Level I STANDING UP, and when you come to an ***** add a march with a hop for 30 seconds.

LEVEL III

TOTAL TIME: 8 minutes

Do Level I STANDING UP, and when you come to an ***** add a march with a hop, swinging arms for 1 minute.

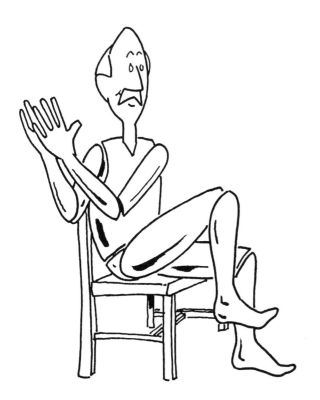

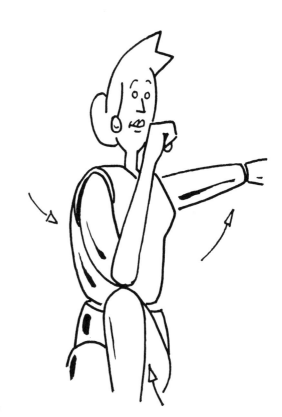

BODY OF THE CLASS: LET'S TONE UP!

SESSION 1 - LEVEL I
UPPER BACK SQUEEZE: Sets:1

Imagine that a large elastic band is attached to your wrists and is pulling your arms forward — pull against this force!

1. Stretch arms out to the side at shoulder level.

2. Pull your arms back (remember the elastic band), squeezing your shoulder blades together (count 1,2,3).

3. Slowly return to starting position (count 1,2,3).

4. Do this sequence 4 times.

5. Rest.

6. Complete the required number of sets.

LEVEL II
UPPER BACK SQUEEZE: Sets: 1

With your weights around your wrists, do Level I.

LEVEL III
UPPER BACK SQUEEZE: Sets: 1

With your weights around your wrists, do Level I.

Remember:

- do not arch back

- keep this movement slow and smooth

- do not forget to breathekeep knees slightly bent when doing this exercise

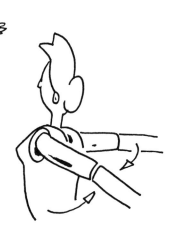

BODY OF THE CLASS: LET'S TONE UP!

SESSION 1 - LEVEL I
BICEP CURLS: Sets: 1

1. Stretch arms out in front of body, palms up.

2. While breathing out, slowly bring hands forward to touch shoulders keeping elbows still (as if to lift a heavy object) (count 1,2,3).

3. While breathing in, slowly return to starting position (count 1,2,3).

4. Lower arms alongside body, stretch arms to the back, slowly lifting hands toward the ceiling (count 1,2,3).

5. Slowly return to starting position (count 1,2,3).

6. Do this sequence 4 times.

7. Rest.

8. Complete the required number of sets.

LEVEL II
BICEP CURLS: Sets: 1

With your weights around your wrists, do Level I .

LEVEL III
BICEP CURLS: Sets: 1

With your weights around your wrists, do Level I .

Remember:

- do not arch back

- keep this movement slow and smooth

- keep knees slightly bent when doing this exercise

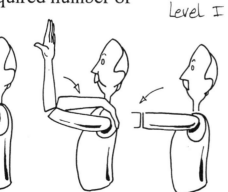

Level I

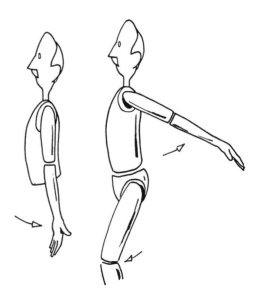

BODY OF THE CLASS: LET'S TONE UP!

SESSION 1 - LEVEL I
BASIC CURL UPS: Sets: 1

1. Lie on your back, bend knees with legs supported on the seat of a chair.

2. Place hands on thighs.

3. While breathing out, slowly raise head and both shoulder blades slightly off the floor (count 1,2,3).

4. While breathing in, slowly lower shoulders to the floor (count 1,2,3).

5. Do this sequence 2 times.

6. Rest.

7. Complete the required number of sets.

LEVEL II
BASIC CURL UPS: Sets: 1

1. Lie on your back, bend knees toward chest, feet off the floor.

2. Place hands on thighs.

3. While breathing out, slowly raise head and both shoulder blades slightly off the floor (count 1,2,3).

4. While breathing in, slowly lower shoulders to the floor (count 1,2,3).

5. Do this sequence 2 times.

6. Rest.

7. Complete the required number of sets.

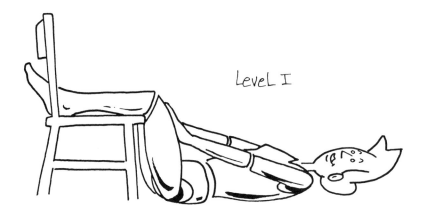

Level I

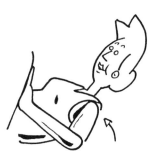

LEVEL III
BASIC CURL UPS: Sets: 1

1. Lie on your back, bend knees with feet flat on the floor.

2. Cross arms and place hands on shoulders.

3. While breathing out, slowly raise head and both shoulder blades slightly off the floor (count 1,2,3).

4. While breathing in, slowly lower shoulders to the floor (count 1,2,3).

5. Do this sequence 2 times.

6. Rest.

7. Complete the required number of sets.

Remember:
- make sure that shoulders touch the floor after each curl up
- raise *both* shoulder blades
- if you have difficulty keeping your feet on the floor, place weights around your ankles
- do not attempt to do a full sit up

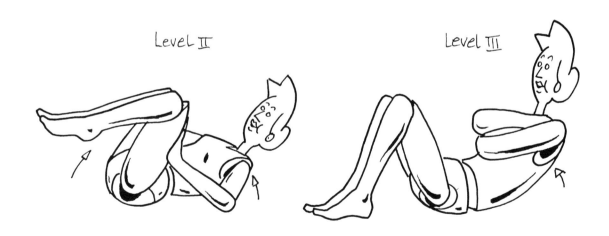

Level II   Level III

BODY OF THE CLASS: LET'S TONE UP!

SESSION 1 - LEVEL I
PELVIC TILT: Sets: 1

1. Lie on your back, bend knees with feet flat on the floor.

2. Tilt your pelvis to press lower back into the floor (count 1,2,3) (tighten your bottom and abdomen).

3. Relax.

4. Do this sequence 2 times.

5. Rest.

6. Complete the required number of sets.

LEVEL II
PELVIC TILT: Sets: 1

1. Lie on your back, bend knees with feet flat on the floor.

2. Tilt your pelvis to press lower back into the floor (tighten your bottom and abdomen).

3. Lift your bottom slightly off the floor keeping lower back on the floor (count 1,2,3).

4. Return to starting position.

5. Do this sequence 2 times.

6. Rest.

7. Complete the required number of sets.

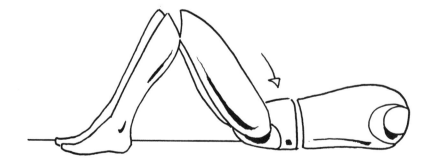

LEVEL III
PELVIC TILT: Sets: 1

1. Lie on your back, bend knees with feet flat on the floor.

2. Tilt your pelvis to press lower back into the floor (tighten your bottom and abdomen).

3. Slowly straighten legs (keep lower back on the floor).

4. When you feel your lower back start to come off the floor, press down on lower back (count 1,2,3).

5. Return to original position.

6. Do this sequence 2 times.

7. Rest.

8. Complete the required number of sets.

Remember:

- keep this movement slow and smooth

- do not forget to breathe

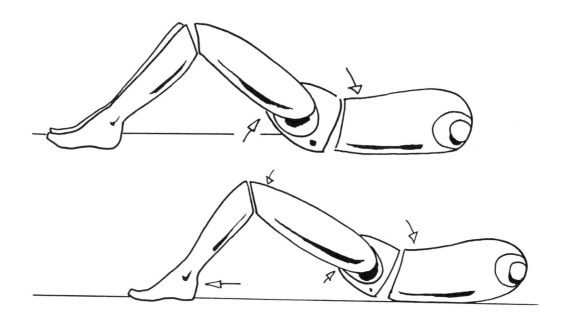

BODY OF THE CLASS: LET'S TONE UP!

SESSION 1 - LEVEL I
LEG TIGHTENERS: Sets: 1

1. Sit down on the floor with back straight and legs outstretched.
2. Place hands on floor behind you.
3. Tighten thigh muscles in both legs (count 1,2,3).
4. Relax.
5. Do this sequence 2 times.
6. Rest.
7. Complete the required number of sets.

LEVEL II
LEG TIGHTENERS: Sets: 2

1. Sit down on the floor with back straight and legs outstretched.
2. Place hands on floor behind you.
3. Tighten thigh muscles in both legs (count 1,2,3).
4. Relax.
5. Do this sequence 4 times.
6. Rest.
7. Complete the required number of sets.

LEVEL III
LEG TIGHTENERS: Sets: 3

1. Sit down on the floor with back straight and legs outstretched.
2. Place hands on floor behind you.
3. Tighten thigh muscles in both legs (count 1,2,3).
4. Relax.
5. Do this sequence 6 times.
6. Rest.
7. Complete the required number of sets.

Remember:
- do not forget to breathe

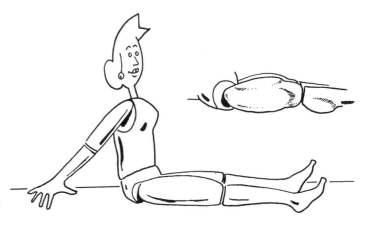

BODY OF THE CLASS: LET'S TONE UP!

SESSION 1 - LEVEL I
SIDE LEG LIFTS: Sets: 1

1. Lie on your left side, head resting on left arm, legs in straight line with your upper body.

2. With toes pointed, slowly lift your right leg as high as possible, keeping hips facing forward (count 1,2,3).

3. Slowly lower right leg to rest on left leg (count 1,2,3).

4. Do this sequence 2 times.

5. Rest.

6. Complete the required number of sets.

7. Turn over so that you lie on your right side.

8. Repeat this exercise with your left leg.

LEVEL II
SIDE LEG LIFTS: Sets: 1

With your weights around your ankles, do Level I.

LEVEL III
SIDE LEG LIFTS: Sets: 1

With your weights around your ankles, do Level I.
Remember:

- do not arch back
- keep upper body still when lifting leg
- use hand on floor in front of you for support
- keep this movement slow and smooth
- do not forget to breathe

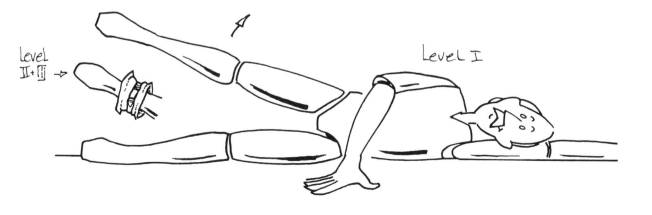

COOL-DOWN: LET'S STRETCH!

SESSION 1 - LEVEL I
SIDE BENDS:

1. Slowly slide right hand down right side of your body, arms relaxed.

2. Tilt head toward right shoulder.

3. Hold this position for 4 seconds.

4. Slowly return to **BASIC POSITION.**

5. Repeat this exercise to the left side.

6. Do this sequence 1 time.

LEVEL II
SIDE BENDS:

1. Lift left arm to the side, bend arm so that elbow is at shoulder height and forearm is hanging down loosely.

2. Slowly slide right hand down right side of your body.

3. Tilt head toward right shoulder.

4. Hold this position for 4 seconds.

5. Slowly return to **BASIC POSITION.**

6. Repeat this exercise to the left side.

7. Do this sequence 2 times.

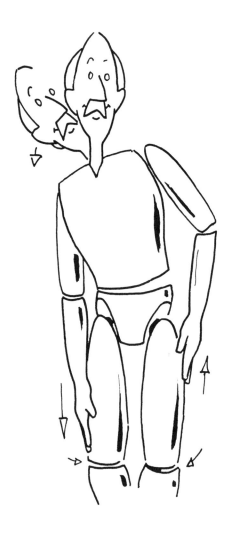

LEVEL III
SIDE BENDS:

1. Put your left hand on your left shoulder, elbow up.

2. Slowly slide right hand down right side of your body.

3. Tilt head toward right shoulder.

4. Hold this position for 5 seconds.

5. Slowly return to **BASIC POSITION**.

6. Repeat this exercise to the left side.

7. Do this sequence 2 times.

Remember:

- do not arch back
- keep knees slightly bent when doing this exercise
- do this exercise slowly
- always bend directly to the side, not forward or backward
- keep hips facing forward
- this exercise can be done while sitting on a chair or with your back against the wall

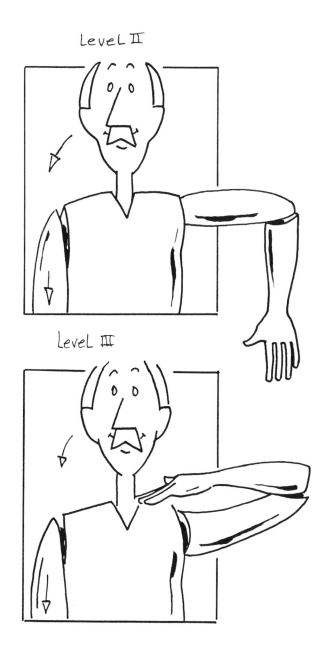

Level II

Level III

COOL-DOWN: LET'S STRETCH!

SESSION 1 - LEVEL I
HUGS:

1. Roll your shoulders forward as far as possible.

2. Turn your head slowly to the right.

3. Hold this position for 4 seconds.

4. Keeping your head to the right, roll your shoulders back as far as possible.

5. Hold this position for 4 seconds.

6. Return to **BASIC POSITION**.

7. Repeat this exercise turning head to left.

8. Do this sequence 1 time.

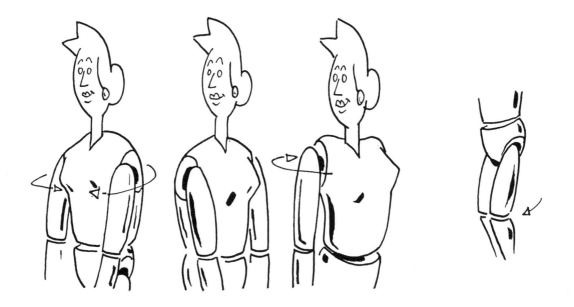

LEVEL II
HUGS:

1. Give yourself a hug, crossing your bent arms in front of you, your hands making fists.

2. Turn your head to look over your right shoulder.

3. Stretch and hold this position for 4 seconds.

4. Keeping your head to the right, uncross arms and bring them behind your body at shoulder level keeping elbows high.

5. Stretch and hold this position for 4 seconds.

6. Return to **BASIC POSITION.**

7. Repeat this exercise, turning head to the left.

8. Do this sequence 2 times.

LEVEL III
HUGS:

1. Give yourself a hug, crossing your bent arms in front of you, your hands making fists.

2. Turn your head to look over your right shoulder.

3. Stretch and hold this position for 5 seconds.

4. Keeping your head to the right, uncross arms and bring them behind your body at shoulder level keeping elbows high.

5. Stretch and hold this position for 5 seconds.

6. Return to **BASIC POSITION.**

7. Repeat this exercise, turning head to the left.

8. Do this sequence 2 times.

Remember:
- do not arch back
- keep knees slightly bent when doing this exercise
- do this exercise slowly
- this exercise can be done while sitting on a chair or with your back against the wall

COOL-DOWN: LET'S STRETCH!

SESSION 1 - LEVEL I
LUNGES:

1. Facing wall at arm's length, keep arms stretched and place palms flat on the wall.

2. Take a step backward with your right leg and place right heel on the floor.

3. Bend your left knee so that it is in line with your toes, bending arms slightly (feel the stretch in your calf muscle!).

4. Hold this position for 4 seconds.

5. Return to starting position.

6. Repeat this exercise with left leg.

7. Do this sequence 1 time.

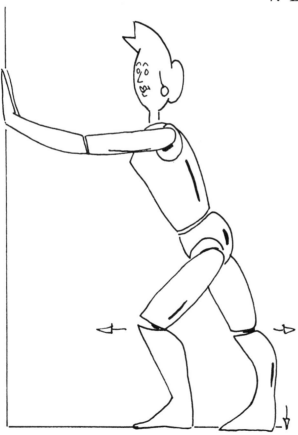

LEVEL II **LUNGES:**	**LEVEL III** **LUNGES:**

LEVEL II
LUNGES:

1. Facing wall at arm's length, keep arms stretched and place palms flat on the wall.

2. Take a step backward with your right leg and place right heel on the floor.

3. Bend your left knee so that it is in line with your toes, bending arms slightly (feel the stretch in your calf muscle!).

4. Hold this position for 4 seconds.

5. Return to starting position.

6. Repeat this exercise with left leg.

7. Do this sequence 2 times.

LEVEL III
LUNGES:

1. Facing wall at arm's length, keep arms stretched and place palms flat on the wall.

2. Take a step backward with your right leg and place right heel on the floor.

3. Bend your left knee so that it is in line with your toes, bending arms slightly (feel the stretch in your calf muscle!).

4. Hold this position for 5 seconds.

5. Return to starting position.

6. Repeat this exercise with left leg.

7. Do this sequence 2 times.

Remember:
- be sure that your knee stays in line with your toes
- do this exercise slowly

COOL-DOWN: LET'S STRETCH!

SESSION 1 - LEVEL I
TURN AROUNDS:

1. Keeping hips still, turn upper body to the right.

2. Look over your right shoulder.

3. Hold this position for 4 seconds.

4. Return to **BASIC POSITION**.

5. Repeat this exercise to the left side.

6. Do this sequence 1 time.

LEVEL II
TURN AROUNDS:

1. Place arms in front of your body at shoulder level, elbows bent, hands on forearms.

2. Keeping hips still, slowly turn upper body to the right, looking over your right shoulder.

3. Reach and hold this position for 4 seconds.

4. Return to starting position.

5. Repeat this exercise to the left side.

6. Do this sequence 2 times.

Level I

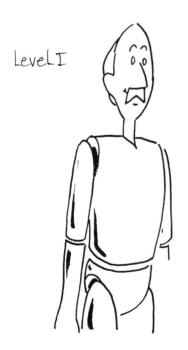
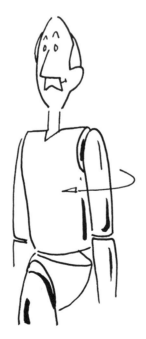
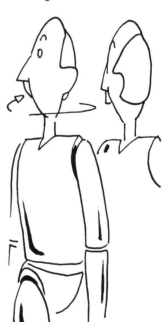

LEVEL III
TURN AROUNDS:

1. Place arms straight out in front of your body at shoulder level.

2. Slowly turn upper body to the right, looking over your right shoulder, swinging both arms slowly to the back at shoulder level.

3. Reach and hold this position for 5 seconds.

4. Return to starting position.

5. Repeat this exercise to the left side.

6. Do this sequence 2 times.

Remember:
- do not force these positions
- do this exercise slowly and smoothly
- always keep knees slightly bent
- keep hips facing forward

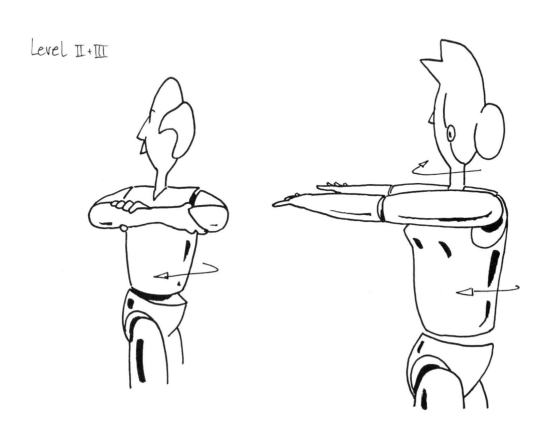

Level II + III

COOL-DOWN: LET'S RELAX!

SESSION 1 - LEVEL I

READ THE COMPLETE
RELAXATION EXERCISE
BEFORE YOU BEGIN

This relaxation should take
approximately 4 minutes to complete.

1. Turn on soft background music.

2. Lie on your back and cover
   yourself with a warm blanket.

3. Listen to the music and let your
   body relax.

4. Imagine that the music is entering
   your body through your toes and is
   flowing to your head.

5. Breathe slowly until your body is
   completely relaxed.

6. Let this relaxed feeling flow
   through your body — ENJOY.

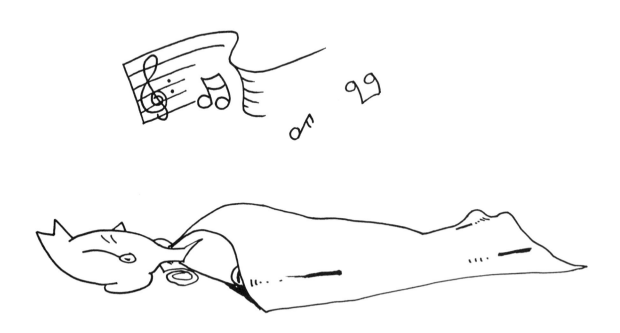

LEVEL II

Do Level I

LEVEL III

Do Level I.

Remember:

- if possible, turn off some of the lights where you will be relaxing

- relax in a quiet area

- keep your breathing slow and rhythmic

- close your eyes when relaxing

- if you have a sleeping bag, use it rather than a blanket — it is excellent for these exercises

- be aware of the difference in your muscles when they are tensed or relaxed

- use a towel or a small pillow at the nape of your neck for support

- if you have lower back problems, support your legs on the seat of a chair

LET'S GET FIT - SESSION 2

WARM-UP: LET'S BEGIN!

SESSION 2 - LEVEL I

TOTAL TIME: 4 minutes

PUT ON SOME LIVELY MUSIC.

SIT ON A CHAIR, FEET FLAT ON THE FLOOR. MAKE SURE THAT YOUR BACK AND BOTTOM ARE TOUCHING THE BACK OF THE CHAIR.

1. Walk on the spot at a slow relaxed pace for 30 seconds.

2. Continue to walk on the spot and do the following movements for 30 seconds each:

a) lean head from side to side

b) swing arms forward and backward, crossing arms in front and behind body

c) walk on the balls of your feet

d) walk on your heels

e) lift knees and clap hands under lifted knee

f) kick in front

g) gradually, step more slowly

3. Stretch both arms above your head and breathe in deeply (2 times).

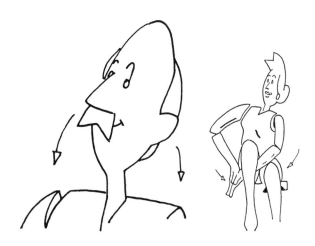

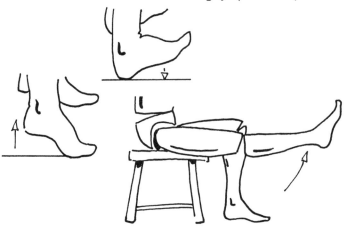

LEVEL II	LEVEL III
Do Level I STANDING UP.	Do Level I STANDING UP.

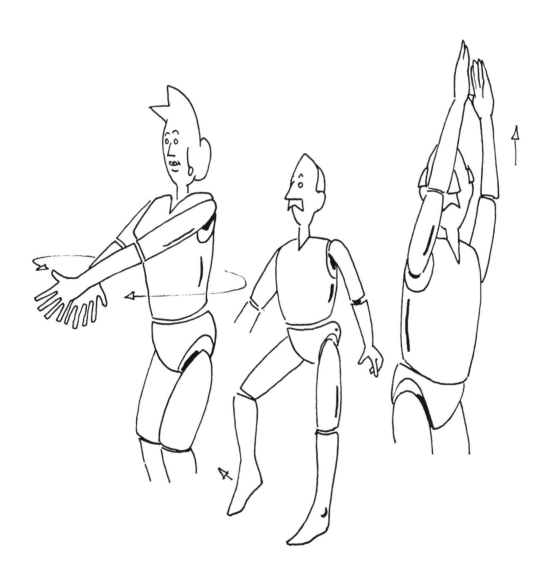

WARM-UP: LET'S LOOSEN UP!

SESSION 2 - LEVEL I
LOOK AROUNDS:

1. Clasp your hands in front of your chest, elbows up.

2. Keeping hands clasped, raise arms above your head, raising your head to keep looking at your hands (you should feel the stretch in your neck).

3. Return to starting position.

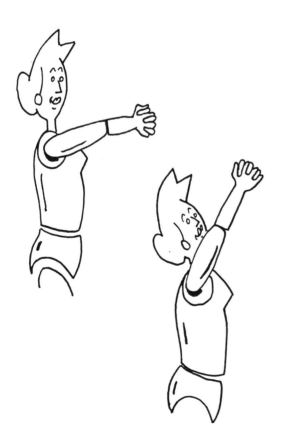

4. Stretch arms to right, turning head to the right.

5. Repeat this movement to the opposite side.

6. Return to starting position.

7. Do this sequence 4 times.

LEVEL II
LOOK AROUNDS:

1. Clasp your hands in front of your chest, elbows up.

2. Keeping hands clasped, raise arms above your head, raising your head to keep looking at your hands (you should feel the stretch in your neck).

3. Return to starting position.

4. Stretch arms to the right, turning head to the left.

5. Repeat this movement to the opposite side.

6. Return to starting position.

7. Do this sequence 4 times.

LEVEL III
LOOK AROUNDS:

1. Clasp your hands in front of your chest, elbows up.

2. Keeping hands clasped, raise arms above your head, raising your head to keep looking at your hands (you should feel the stretch in your neck).

3. Return to starting position.

4. Stretch arms to the right, turning head to the left.

5. Repeat this movement to the opposite side.

6. Return to starting position.

7. Do this sequence 6 times.

Remember:

- do not arch back
- do not tip head backward
- keep hips still
- do not force this movement

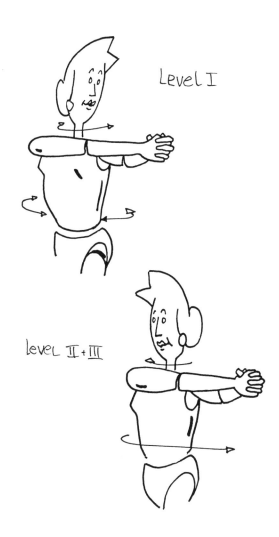

Level I

level II + III

WARM-UP: LET'S LOOSEN UP!

SESSION 2 - LEVEL I
BLINKS:

1. Exaggerate blinking; keep your eyes closed tightly.

2. Open eyes wide, pulling your chin downward.

3. Relax.

4. Do this sequence 4 times.

LEVEL II
BLINKS:

1. Exaggerate blinking; keep your eyes closed tightly.

2. Open your eyes wide, pulling your chin downward.

3. Relax.

4. Exaggerate a frown, keep this frown and wink on the right side.

5. Frown again and wink on the left side.

6. Relax.

7. Do this sequence 4 times.

LEVEL III
BLINKS:

1. Exaggerate blinking; keep your eyes closed tightly.

2. Open your eyes wide, pulling your chin downward.

3. Relax.

4. Exaggerate a frown; keep this frown and wink on the right side.

5. Frown again and wink on the left side.

6. Relax.

7. Do this sequence 6 times.

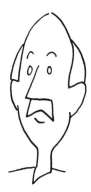 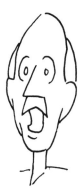 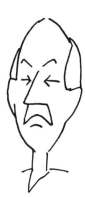 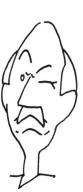

WARM-UP: LET'S LOOSEN UP!

SESSION 2 - LEVEL I
SHOULDER ROLLS:

1. Moving both shoulders at the same time, raise shoulders and move them forward, down, back and up, in a circular motion.

2. Complete 4 circles.

3. Reverse moving shoulders up, back, down and front.

LEVEL II
SHOULDER ROLLS:

1. Place hands on shoulders.

2. Moving both elbows at the same time, slowly describe 4 circles with your elbows, moving forward, down, back and up.

3. Reverse.

LEVEL III
SHOULDER ROLLS:

1. Place hands on shoulders.

2. Moving both elbows at the same time, slowly describe 6 circles with your elbows, moving forward, down, back and up.

3. Reverse.

Remember:

- do not arch back
- keep a slow, smooth rhythm

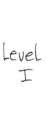

Level I

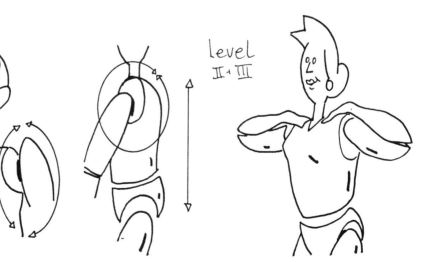

Level II + III

WARM-UP: LET'S LOOSEN UP!

SESSION 2 - LEVEL I
DOUBLE CIRCLES:

1. Clasp hands in front of body, elbows down.

2. Keeping hands together, describe 4 large circles.

3. Repeat in opposite direction.

LEVEL II
DOUBLE CIRCLES:

1. Place palm against palm in front of body, fingers extended and pointing up, elbows down.

2. Keeping palms together, describe 4 large circles with your hands.

3. Repeat in opposite direction.

LEVEL III
DOUBLE CIRCLES:

1. Place palm against palm in front of body, fingers extended and pointing up, elbows down.

2. Keeping palms together, describe 6 large circles with your hands.

3. Repeat in opposite direction.

Remember:

- keep elbows and forearms still

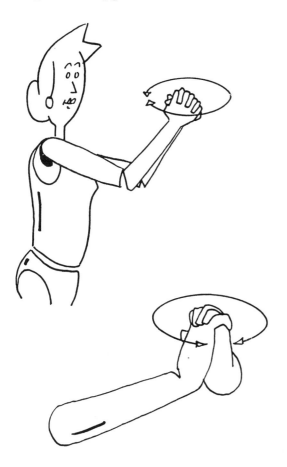

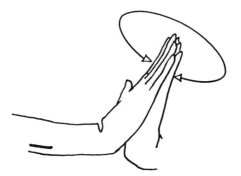

WARM-UP: LET'S LOOSEN UP!

SESSION 2 - LEVEL I
CAT SCRATCHES:

1. Spread your fingers on both hands as far apart as possible.

2. Make a scratch like a cat sharpening its claws.

3. Make fists with both hands.

4. Relax hands and shake them out.

5. Do this sequence 4 times.

LEVEL II
CAT SCRATCHES:

1. Spread your fingers on both hands as far apart as possible.

2. Bend your fingers to touch the heels of your hands with a cat-like scratching movement.

3. Spread your fingers as far apart as possible.

4. Do this sequence 4 times.

LEVEL III
CAT SCRATCHES:

1. Spread your fingers on both hands as far apart as possible.

2. Bend your fingers to touch the heels of your hands with a cat-like scratching movement.

3. Spread your fingers as far apart as possible.

4. Do this sequence 6 times.

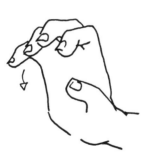

Level I

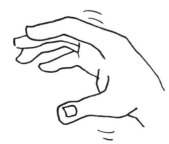

Level II + III

WARM-UP: LET'S LOOSEN UP!

SESSION 2 - LEVEL I
KNEE SWINGS:

1. Sit down on the floor, back straight.

2. Bend knees toward your chest, feet together on the floor.

3. Place hands on the floor beside you, fingers pointing sideways.

4. Slowly swing knees to the floor on your right side.

5. Repeat on the other side.

6. Do this sequence 4 times.

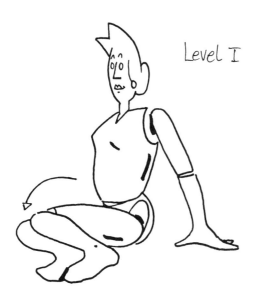

Level I

LEVEL II
KNEE SWINGS:

1. Sit down on the floor, back straight, knees slightly bent, feet together and on the floor.

2. Place hands on the floor beside you, fingers pointing sideways.

3. Cross left leg over right leg.

4. Keeping legs crossed, swing knees to right side, trying to touch the floor.

5. Return to starting position.

6. Repeat exercise, crossing right leg over left and swinging knees to left side.

7. Return to starting position.

8. Do this sequence 4 times.

LEVEL III
KNEE SWINGS:

1. Sit down on the floor, back straight, knees slightly bent, feet together and on the floor.

2. Place hands on the floor beside you, fingers pointing sideways.

3. Cross left leg over right leg.

4. Keeping legs crossed, swing knees to right side, trying to touch the floor.

5. Return to starting position.

6. Repeat exercise, crossing right leg over left and swinging knees to left side.

7. Return to starting position.

8. Do this sequence 6 times.

Remember:
- leave your hands on the floor

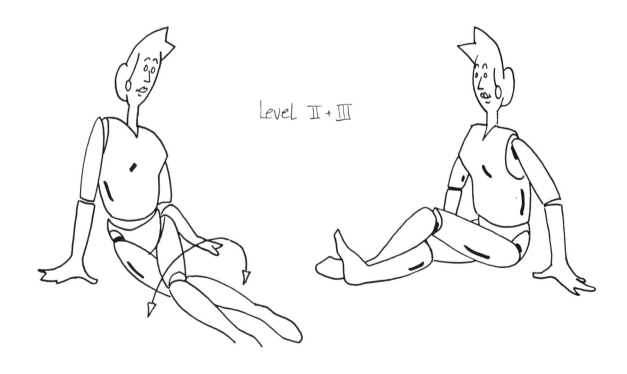

Level II + III

WARM-UP: LET'S LOOSEN UP!

SESSION 2 - LEVEL I
FLOOR CIRCLES:

1. Stand with left side toward the wall at arm's length. Place palm flat against the wall at shoulder height.

2. Stretch right leg forward with toes pointed, keeping toes on the floor.

3. Describe a semicircle with your foot bringing it from the front to the back.

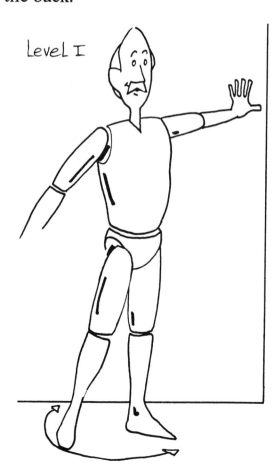

Level I

4. Repeat movement bringing leg from back to front.

5. Do this sequence 4 times.

6. Turn around, place opposite hand on wall.

7. Repeat exercise with left leg.

LEVEL II
FLOOR CIRCLES:

1. Stand with left side toward the wall at arm's length. Place palm flat against the wall at shoulder height.

2. Lift right leg up in front at knee height, toes pointed.

3. Describe a semicircle with your leg bringing it from the front to the back.

4. Repeat movement bringing leg from back to front.

5. Return to starting position.

6. Do this sequence 4 times.

7. Turn around, place opposite hand on wall.

8. Repeat exercise with left leg.

LEVEL III
FLOOR CIRCLES:

1. Stand with left side toward the wall at arm's length. Place palm flat against the wall at shoulder height.

2. Lift right leg up in front at knee height, toes pointed.

3. Describe a semicircle with your leg bringing it from the front to the back.

4. Repeat movement bringing leg from back to front.

5. Return to starting position.

6. Do this sequence 6 times.

7. Turn around, place opposite hand on wall.

8. Repeat exercise with left leg.

Remember:

- do not arch your back
- do not put weight on pointing foot
- do not over cross when your leg is in the back

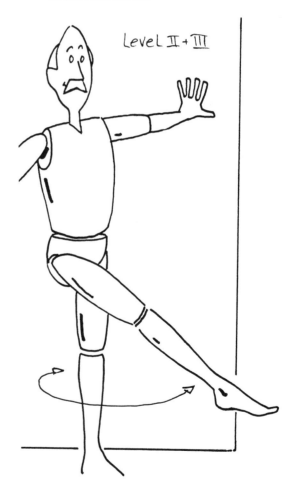

Level II + III

WARM-UP: LET'S LOOSEN UP!

SESSION 2 - LEVEL I
TOES SEMICIRCLE:

1. Stand with left side toward the wall at arm's length. Place palm of hand flat against the wall at shoulder height.

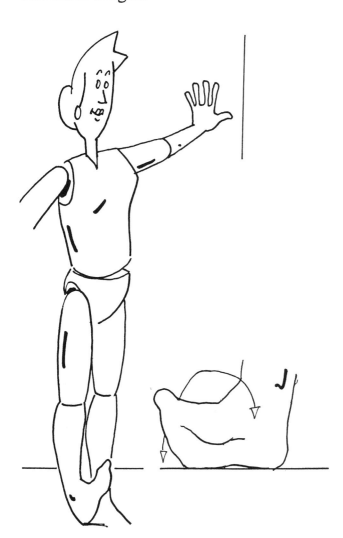

2. Keeping heel on the floor, describe a semicircle by swinging toes of your right foot to the side.

3. Return to starting position.

4. Do this sequence 4 times.

5. Turn around, place opposite hand on wall.

6. Repeat exercise with left foot.

LEVEL II
TOES SEMICIRCLE:

1. Sit on the floor, back straight, knees bent toward your chest, feet flat on floor, shoulder-width apart.

2. Flex both feet so that toes are pointing toward the ceiling.

3. Keeping heels on floor, describe a semicircle by swinging toes to the outside, trying to touch the outside of your feet to the floor.

4. Return to starting position.

5. Do this sequence 4 times.

LEVEL III
TOES SEMICIRCLE:

1. Sit on the floor, back straight, knees bent toward your chest, feet flat on floor, shoulder-width apart.

2. Flex both feet so that toes are pointing toward the ceiling.

3. Keeping heels on floor, describe a semicircle by swinging toes to the outside, trying to touch the outside of your feet to the floor.

4. Return to starting position.

5. Do this sequence 6 times.

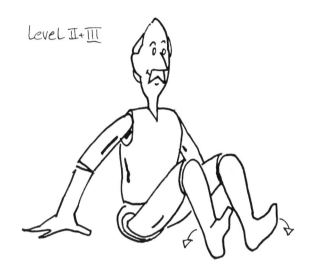

Level II+III

BODY OF THE CLASS: LET'S ENERGIZE!

SESSION 2 - LEVEL I

TOTAL TIME: 5 minutes

PUT ON SOME UPBEAT MUSIC.

SIT ON A CHAIR, FEET FLAT ON THE FLOOR. MAKE SURE THAT YOUR BACK AND BOTTOM ARE TOUCHING THE BACK OF THE CHAIR.

Do the following movements for 30 seconds each:

1. Walk on the spot.

2. March, lifting knees and swinging arms.

   ✱

3. While clapping hands, lift right knee and kick right foot in front. Repeat with left leg.

4. Point right foot in front on the floor. Repeat with left foot.

5. Continue pointing, swing arms above head from side to side.

6. Continue pointing, reach right arm up to ceiling, then left arm.

   ✱

7. Step side to side.

BODY CHECK - SING!

8. Stand up and raise both arms overhead. Sit down. Repeat several times.

9. March, swim with your arms (the crawl).

10. Walk slowly.

11. Tap toes.

Stretch both arms above your head and breathe in deeply (2 times).

BODY CHECK MONITOR HEART RATE!

LEVEL II

TOTAL TIME: 7 minutes

Do Level I STANDING UP, and when you come to an * add a march with a hop for 30 seconds.

LEVEL III

TOTAL TIME: 8 minutes

Do Level I STANDING UP, and when you come to an * add a march with a hop, swinging arms for 1 minute.

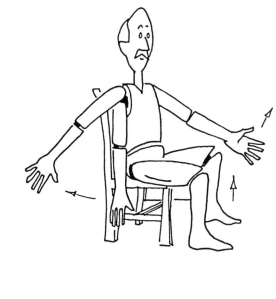

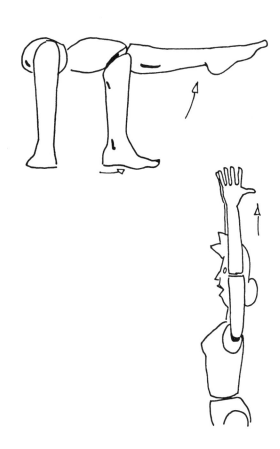

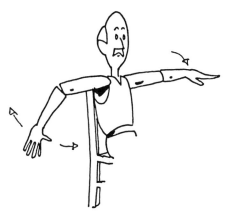

BODY OF THE CLASS: LET'S TONE UP!

SESSION 2 - LEVEL I
ROW BOATS: Sets: 2

Imagine that a large elastic band is attached to your wrists and keeps your arms from pulling backward or forward - pull against this force!

1. Stretch arms out to the side at shoulder level, palms facing back.

2. Spread the fingers of both hands as far apart as you can.

3. Slowly pull your arms backward (remember the elastic band!) (count 1,2,3).

4. Turn palms to face the front, slowly push your arms forward (remember the elastic band!) (count 1,2,3).

5. Do this sequence 5 times.

6. Rest.

7. Complete the required number of sets.

LEVEL II
ROW BOATS: Sets: 2

With your weights around your wrists, do Level I.

LEVEL III
ROW BOATS: Sets: 2

With your weights around your wrists, do Level I.

Remember:

- do not arch back

- keep this movement slow and smooth

- do not forget to breathe

- keep knees slightly bent when doing this exercise

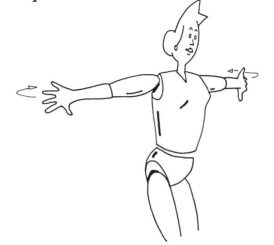

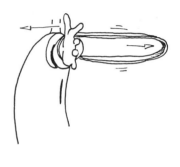

BODY OF THE CLASS: LET'S TONE UP!

SESSION 2 - LEVEL I
THE WEIGHT LIFTER: Sets: 2

1. Stretch arms out in front of body, palms up, make tight fists and...

2. While breathing out, slowly bring hands to touch shoulders keeping elbows still (as if to lift a heavy object) (count 1,2,3).

3. While breathing in, slowly return to starting position (count 1,2,3).

4. Lower arms alongside body and stretch arms to the back, slowly lifting hands toward the ceiling (count 1,2,3).

5. Slowly return to starting position (count 1,2,3).

6. Do this sequence 5 times.

7. Rest.

8. Complete the required number of sets.

LEVEL II
THE WEIGHT LIFTER: Sets:2

With your weights around your wrists, do Level I .

LEVEL III
THE WEIGHT LIFTER: Sets: 2

With your weights around your wrists, do Level I .

Remember:

- do not arch back
- keep this movement slow and smooth
- keep knees slightly bent when doing this exercise

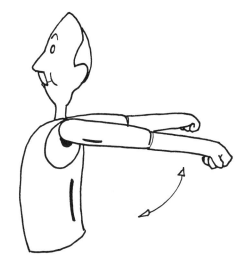

BODY OF THE CLASS: LET'S TONE UP!

SESSION 2 - LEVEL I
CURL UP CROSSOVERS: Sets: 2

1. Lie on your back, bend knees with legs supported on the seat of a chair.

2. Place hands on thighs.

3. While breathing out, slowly raise head and both shoulder blades slightly off the floor and touch the outside of your right knee with your left hand (count 1,2,3).

4. While breathing in, slowly lower shoulders to the floor (count 1,2,3).

5. Repeat this exercise on the other side.

6. Do this sequence 2 times.

7. Rest.

8. Complete the required number of sets.

LEVEL II
CURL UP CROSSOVERS: Sets: 2

1. Lie on your back, bend knees toward chest, feet off the floor.

2. Place hands on thighs.

3. While breathing out, slowly raise head and both shoulder blades slightly off the floor and touch the outside of your right knee with your left hand (count 1,2,3).

4. While breathing in, slowly lower shoulders to the floor (count 1,2,3).

5. Repeat this exercise on the other side.

6. Do this sequence 2 times.

7. Rest.

8. Complete the required number of sets.

Level I

Level II

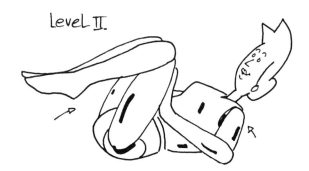

LEVEL III
CURL UP CROSSOVERS: Sets: 2

1. Lie on your back, bend knees with feet flat on the floor.

2. Cross arms and place hands on shoulders.

3. While breathing out, slowly raise head and both shoulder blades slightly off the floor. Try to touch your right knee with your left elbow (count 1,2,3).

4. While breathing in, slowly lower shoulders to the floor (count 1,2,3).

5. Repeat this exercise on the other side.

6. Do this sequence 2 times.

7. Rest.

8. Complete the required number of sets.

Remember:

- make sure that shoulders touch the floor after each curl up

- raise *both* shoulder blades

- if you have difficulty keeping your feet on the floor, place weights around your ankles

- do not attempt to do a full sit up

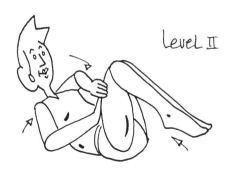

Level II

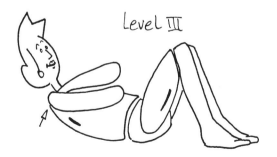

Level III

BODY OF THE CLASS: LET'S TONE UP!

SESSION 2 - LEVEL I
THE SHUFFLE: Sets: 2

1. Sit on the floor, knees slightly bent.

2. Squeeze your bottom tightly (as if you are trying to hold something) (count 1,2,3).

3. Relax.

4. Do this sequence 2 times.

5. Rest.

6. Complete the required number of sets.

LEVEL II
THE SHUFFLE: Sets: 2

1. Sit on the floor, knees slightly bent.

2. Squeeze your bottom tightly and slowly take 4 steps forward (as if you were walking with your bottom).

3. Take 4 steps backward.

4. Relax.

5. Do this sequence 2 times.

6. Rest.

7. Complete the required number of sets.

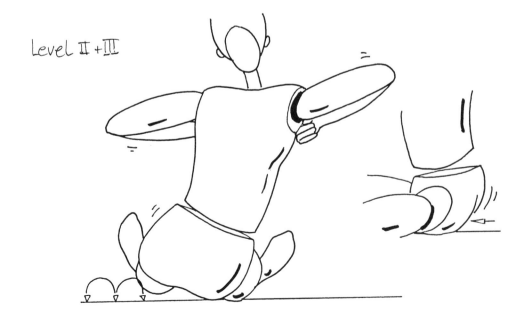

Level II + III

LEVEL III
THE SHUFFLE: Sets: 2

1. Sit on the floor, knees slightly bent.

2. Squeeze your bottom tightly and slowly take 4 steps forward, 4 backward, 4 to the left and 4 to the right.

3. Relax.

4. Do this sequence 2 times.

5. Rest.

6. Complete the required number of sets.

Remember:

- if you have problems with your back, do Level I sitting down with your back against a wall

- keep your shoulders facing forward

BODY OF THE CLASS: LET'S TONE UP!

| SESSION 2 - LEVEL I |
| QUADS TENSE: Sets: 2 |

1. Sit on the floor, back straight, right leg outstretched and left knee bent.

2. Place hands on the floor behind you.

3. Straighten right leg tightening the thigh muscles and lift leg so that heel *slightly* comes off the floor (count 1,2,3).

4. Slowly lower leg to the floor (count 1,2,3).

5. Repeat this exercise with the left leg.

6. Do this sequence 2 times.

7. Rest.

8. Complete the required number of sets.

| LEVEL II |
| QUADS TENSE: Sets: 2 |

With your weights around your ankles, do Level I.

| LEVEL III |
| QUADS TENSE: Sets: 2 |

With your weights around your ankles, do Level I.

Remember:

- do not forget to breathe

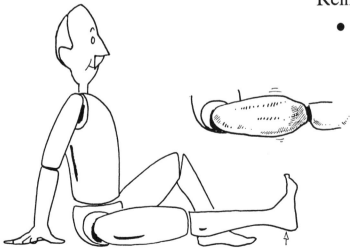

BODY OF THE CLASS: LET'S TONE UP!

SESSION 2 - LEVEL I FLEX SIDE LEG LIFTS: Sets: 2

1. Lie on your left side, head resting on left arm, legs in straight line with your upper body.

2. Flex right foot.

3. Keeping foot flexed, slowly lift your right leg as high as possible, keeping hips facing forward (count 1,2,3).

4. Slowly lower right leg to rest on left leg (count 1,2,3).

5. Do this sequence 2 times.

6. Complete the required number of sets.

7. Turn over so that you lie on your right side.

8. Repeat this exercise with your left leg.

LEVEL II FLEX SIDE LEG LIFTS: Sets: 2

With your weights around your ankles, do Level I.

LEVEL III FLEX SIDE LEG LIFTS: Sets: 2

With your weights around your ankles, do Level I.

Remember:

- do not arch back

- keep upper body still when lifting leg

- use hand on floor in front of you for support

- keep this movement slow and smooth

- do not forget to breathe

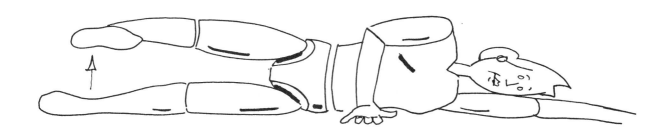

COOL-DOWN: LET'S STRETCH!

SESSION 2 - LEVEL I
REACHES:

1. Stretch right arm toward ceiling, fingers pointing upward. While keeping chin up and looking at lifting arm...

2. Reach as far as possible toward the ceiling with your right arm (feel that stretch!).

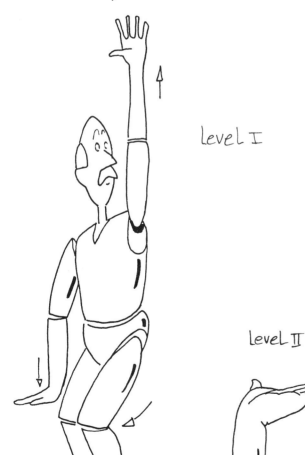

Level I

Level II

3. Hold this position for 4 seconds.

4. Return to **BASIC POSITION**.

5. Repeat this exercise with left arm.

6. Repeat this sequence, keeping arms down and pressing fingers toward the floor.

7. Do this sequence 2 times.

LEVEL II
REACHES:

1. Stretch right arm toward ceiling, wrist flexed and palm facing ceiling. While keeping chin up and looking at lifting arm...

2. Reach as far as possible toward the ceiling with your right arm (feel that stretch!).

3. Hold this position for 4 seconds.

4. Return to **BASIC POSITION**.

5. Repeat this exercise with left arm.

6. Repeat this sequence, keeping arms down and pressing palms of hands toward the floor.

7. Do this sequence 3 times.

LEVEL III
REACHES:

1. Stretch both arms over your head.

2. Cross your arms at the wrists and clasp hands.

3. Stretch hands toward the ceiling.

4. Hold this position for 5 seconds.

5. Return to **BASIC POSITION.**

6. Cross arms at wrists behind back and clasp hands.

7. Stretch arms down toward the floor.

8. Hold this position for 5 seconds.

9. Return to **BASIC POSITION.**

10. Do this sequence 3 times.

Remember:

- do not arch back
- keep knees slightly bent when doing this exercise
- do this exercise slowly
- this exercise can be done while sitting on a chair
- keep hips facing forward

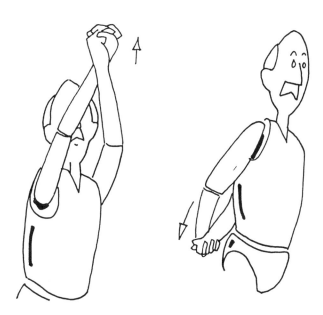
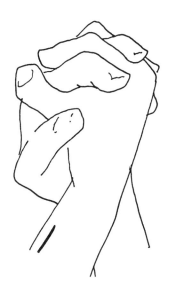

COOL-DOWN: LET'S STRETCH!

SESSION 2 - LEVEL I
FRONT AND BACKS:

1. Slowly raise arms behind your back, keeping arms straight.

2. Reach and hold this position for 4 seconds.

3. Return to **BASIC POSITION**.

4. With arms straight, cross your arms in front of your chest.

5. Reach and hold this position for 4 seconds.

6. Do this sequence 2 times.

LEVEL II
FRONT AND BACKS:

1. Clasp hands behind your back.

2. Pull arms down and hold this position for 4 seconds.

3. Bring arms in front of body at shoulder level, cross arms at wrists and clasp hands.

4. Pull arms forward and hold this position for 4 seconds.

5. Do this sequence 3 times.

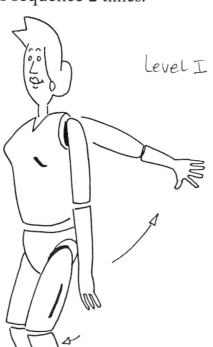

Level I

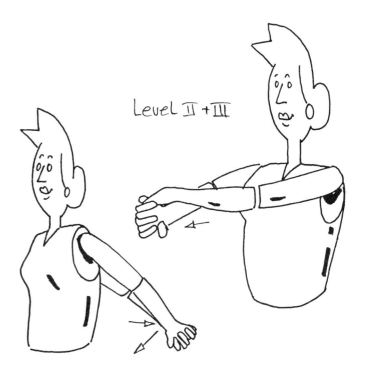

Level II + III

LEVEL III
FRONT AND BACKS:

1. Clasp hands behind your back.

2. Pull hands toward the ceiling.

3. Stretch and hold this position for 5 seconds.

4. Bring arms in front of body at shoulder level, cross arms at wrists and clasp hands.

5. Stretch arms toward the ceiling.

6. Stretch and hold this position for 5 seconds.

7. Do this sequence 3 times.

Remember:

- do not arch back

- keep knees slightly bent when doing this exercise

- do this exercise slowly

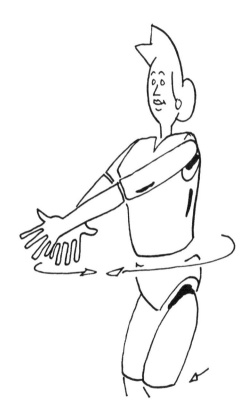

COOL-DOWN: LET'S STRETCH!

SESSION 2 - LEVEL I
BEND AND STRETCH:

1. Lying on left side, bend both knees slightly, right hand in front of body on floor for support.

2. Slowly swing right leg in front of your stomach without touching the floor, keeping knee straight.

3. Flex your right foot.

4. Hold this position for 4 seconds.

5. Slowly swing right leg to the back and bend your knee. Do not arch back!

6. Hold this position for 4 seconds.

7. Return to starting position.

8. Do this sequence 2 times.

9. Change sides and repeat this exercise with left leg.

LEVEL II
BEND AND STRETCH:

1. Lying on left side, bend both knees slightly, right hand in front of body on floor for support.

2. Slowly swing right leg in front of your stomach without touching the floor, keeping knee straight.

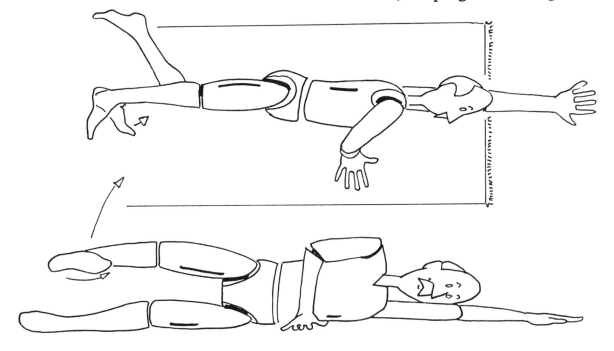

3. Flex your right foot.

4. Hold this position for 4 seconds.

5. Slowly swing right leg to the back and bend your knee. Do not arch back!

6. Hold this position for 4 seconds.

7. Return to starting position.

8. Do this sequence 3 times.

9. Change sides and repeat this exercise with left leg.

LEVEL III
BEND AND STRETCH:

---

1. Lying on left side, bend both knees slightly, right hand in front of body on floor for support.

2. Slowly swing right leg in front of your stomach without touching the floor, keeping knee straight.

3. Flex your right foot.

4. Hold this position for 5 seconds.

5. Slowly swing right leg to the back and bend your knee. Do not arch back!

6. Hold this position for 5 seconds.

7. Return to starting position.

8. Do this sequence 3 times.

9. Change sides and repeat this exercise with left leg.

Remember:

- do this exercise slowly

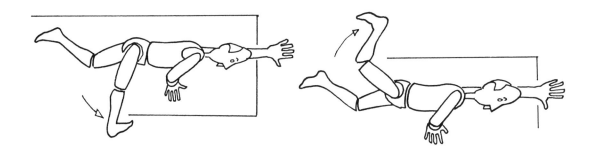

COOL-DOWN: LET'S STRETCH!

SESSION 2 - LEVEL I **WAIST TWISTS:**	**LEVEL II** **WAIST TWISTS:**

1. Keeping hips still, knees slightly bent, turn upper body to the right.

2. Try to touch both hands to the back of your thighs.

3. Reach and hold this position for 4 seconds.

4. Return to **BASIC POSITION.**

5. Repeat this exercise to the left side.

6. Do this sequence 2 times.

1. Place arms in front of your body at shoulder level, elbows bent, hands on forearms.

2. Keeping hips still, slowly turn upper body to the right, looking over your right shoulder, releasing your right arm and slowly swinging it to the back.

3. Reach and hold this position for 4 seconds.

4. Return to starting position.

5. Repeat this exercise to the left side.

6. Do this sequence 3 times.

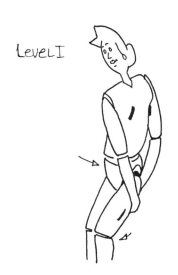

Level I

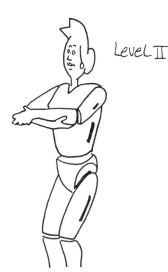

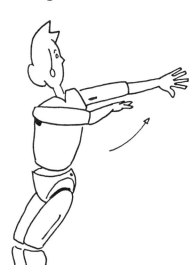

Level II

LEVEL III
WAIST TWISTS:

1. Sit on the floor, knees slightly bent, arms relaxed in front of your body.

2. Turn the upper body to the right and place your hands on the floor behind you.

3. Reach and hold this position for 5 seconds.

4. Return to starting position.

5. Repeat this exercise to the left side.

6. Do this sequence 3 times.

Remember:
- do not force these positions
- do this exercise slowly and smoothly
- always keep your knees slightly bent

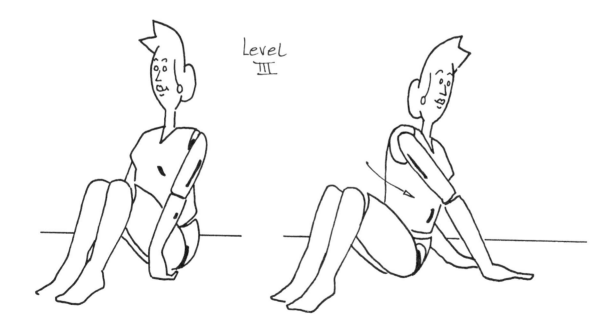

Level III

COOL-DOWN: LET'S RELAX!

SESSION 2 - LEVEL I

READ THE COMPLETE
RELAXATION EXERCISE
BEFORE YOU BEGIN

TOTAL TIME: 4 minutes

1. Turn on soft background music.

2. Lie on your back and cover yourself with a warm blanket.

3. Pretend that your body is becoming so heavy that it is being pulled into the floor.

4. Try to lift your limbs, one at a time (remember, they are too heavy to lift).

5. Breathe slowly until your body is completely relaxed.

6. Let this relaxed feeling flow through your body — ENJOY.

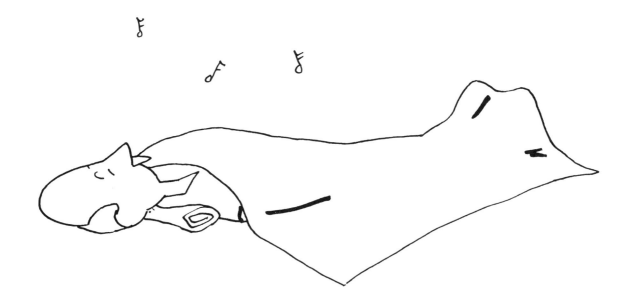

LEVEL II

Do Level I.

LEVEL III

Do Level I.

Remember:

- if possible, turn off some of the lights where you will be relaxing

- relax in a quiet area

- keep your breathing slow and rhythmic

- close your eyes when relaxing

- if you have a sleeping bag, use it rather than a blanket — it is excellent for these exercises

- be aware of the difference in your muscles when they are tensed or relaxed

- use a towel or a small pillow at the nape of your neck for support

- if you have lower back problems support your legs on the seat of a chair

LET'S GET FIT - SESSION 3

WARM-UP: LET'S BEGIN!

SESSION 3 - LEVEL I

TOTAL TIME: 4 minutes

PUT ON SOME LIVELY MUSIC.

1. Point right foot on the floor in front of body, then left foot, at a slow, relaxed pace for 30 seconds.

2. Continue pointing and do the following movements for 30 seconds each:

a) extend right arm in front of body, then left arm

b) swing arms from side to side at shoulder level

c) bend upper body from side to side

d) instead of pointing toes on floor, place heels on floor

e) walk forward crossing legs one in front of the other

f) walk backward, crossing legs one behind the other

g) gradually, step more slowly.

3. Stretch both arms above your head and breathe in deeply (2 times).

LEVEL II	LEVEL III
Do Level I.	Do Level I.

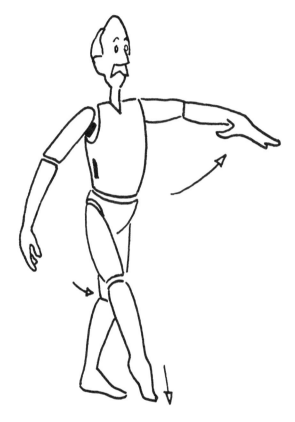

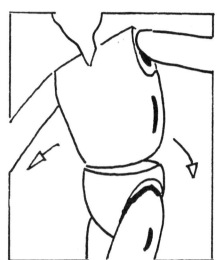

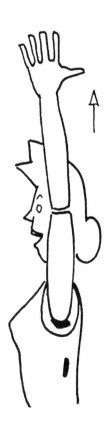

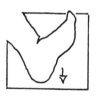

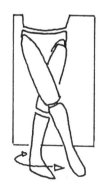

WARM-UP: LET'S LOOSEN UP!

SESSION 3 - LEVEL I
SIDE TO SIDES:

1. Lean head toward the right, bringing the ear toward the shoulder while looking ahead.

2. Return to centre.

3. Repeat, leaning head to the left side.

4. Do this sequence 4 times.

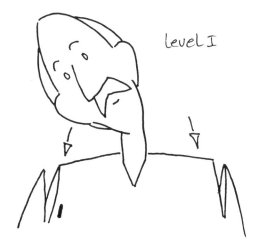

level I

LEVEL II
SIDE TO SIDES:

1. Place arms down along sides of body, press heels of hands toward the floor. Keep this tension in your arms and...

2. Lean head toward the right, bringing the ear toward your shoulder while looking ahead. Press heel of left hand further toward the floor.

3. Return to starting position.

4. Repeat, leaning head to left side, pressing right hand toward the floor.

5. Do this sequence 4 times.

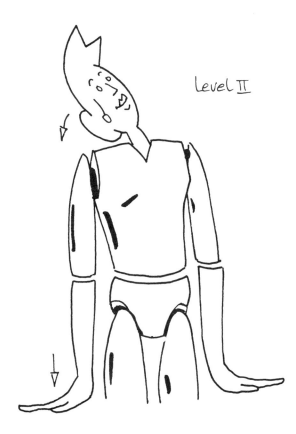

level II

LEVEL III
SIDE TO SIDES:

1. Place arms down along sides of body, press heels of hands towards the floor. Keep this tension in your arms and...

2. Lean head toward the right, bringing the ear toward your shoulder while looking ahead. Press heel of left hand further toward the floor.

3. Return to starting position.

4. Repeat, leaning head to left side, pressing right hand toward the floor.

5. Do this sequence 6 times.

Remember:

- do not arch back
- keep shoulders still

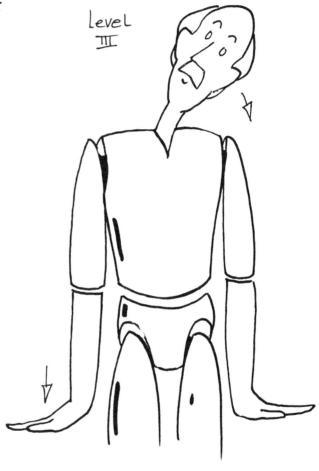

Level III

WARM-UP: LET'S LOOSEN UP!

SESSION 3 - LEVEL I
CHEWS:

1. Keeping your chin up, place your tongue on the roof of your mouth.

2. Exaggerate chewing the air without grinding your teeth.

3. Do this sequence 4 times.

LEVEL II
CHEWS:

1. Keeping your chin up, place your tongue on the roof of your mouth.

2. Exaggerate chewing the air without grinding your teeth.

3. Open your mouth as wide as possible.

4. Do this sequence 4 times.

LEVEL III
CHEWS:

1. Keeping your chin up, place your tongue on the roof of your mouth.

2. Exaggerate chewing the air without grinding your teeth.

3. Open your mouth as wide as possible.

4. Do this sequence 6 times.

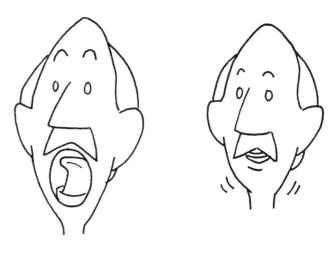

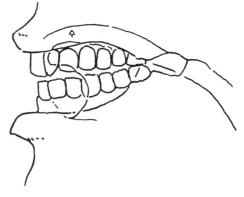

WARM-UP: LET'S LOOSEN UP!

SESSION 3 - LEVEL I
AROUND THE WORLD:

1. Fold your arms in front of your body, hands on forearms.

2. Describe a circle in front of your body with folded arms.

3. Do this sequence 4 times.

4. Repeat in opposite direction.

LEVEL II
AROUND THE WORLD:

1. Stretch your arms in front of your body—arms straight, hands clasped.

2. Describe a large circle with arms outstretched in front of body.

3. Do this sequence 4 times.

4. Repeat in opposite direction.

LEVEL III
AROUND THE WORLD:

1. Stretch your arms in front of your body—arms straight, hands clasped.

2. Describe a large circle with arms outstretched in front of body.

3. Do this sequence 6 times.

4. Repeat in opposite direction.

Remember:

- keep circles in front of body

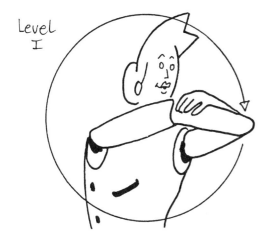

Level I

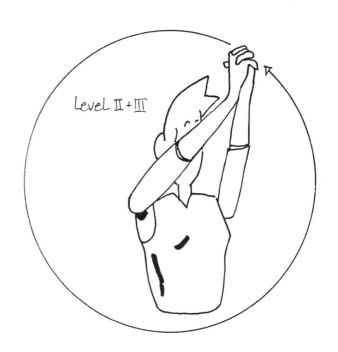

Level II + III

WARM-UP: LET'S LOOSEN UP!

SESSION 3 - LEVEL I
AROUND AND AROUND:

1. Clasp hands in front of body, arms bent, elbows down.

2. Keeping hands together, describe 4 large figure 8s .

3. Repeat in opposite direction.

LEVEL II
AROUND AND AROUND:

1. Place palm against palm in front of body, fingers extended and pointing up, arms bent, elbows down.

2. Keeping palms together, describe 4 large figure 8s with your hands.

3. Repeat in opposite direction.

LEVEL III
AROUND AND AROUND:

1. Place palm against palm in front of body, fingers extended and pointing up, arms bent, elbows down.

2. Keeping palms together, describe 6 large figure-8s with your hands.

3. Repeat in opposite direction.

Remember:

- keep elbows and forearms still

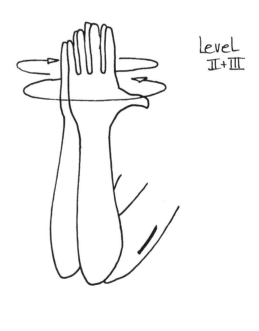

Level II + III

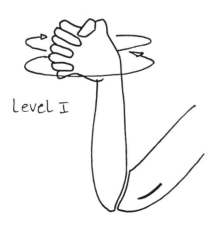

Level I

WARM UP: LET'S LOOSEN UP!

SESSION 3 - LEVEL I
FINGER BENDS:

1. Spread your fingers on both hands as far apart as possible.

2. With both hands, bend the 2 top finger joints as far as you can without closing your hand.

3. Stretch fingers.

4. Do this sequence 4 times.

LEVEL II
FINGER BENDS:

1. Spread your fingers on both hands as far apart as possible.

2. With both hands, bend the 2 top finger joints so that the tips of your fingers try to touch the bottoms of the same fingers.

3. Stretch fingers.

4. Do this sequence 4 times.

LEVEL III
FINGER BENDS:

1. Spread your fingers on both hands as far apart as possible.

2. With both hands, bend the 2 top finger joints so that the tips of your fingers try to touch the bottoms of the same fingers.

3. Stretch fingers.

4. Do this sequence 6 times.

Remember:

- keep wrists still
- keep movements slow and smooth
- do not force this movement

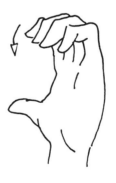
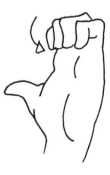

WARM-UP: LET'S LOOSEN UP!

SESSION 3 - LEVEL I
ROLL OVERS:

1. Lie on your back, knees bent, feet on the floor, arms outstretched at shoulder level.

2. Slowly swing knees to your right side until they touch the floor, releasing left shoulder from the floor.

3. Repeat, swinging knees to left side.

4. Do this sequence 4 times.

LEVEL II
ROLL OVERS:

1. Lie on your back, knees slightly bent, arms outstretched at shoulder level.

2. Lifting feet off the floor, bring your knees toward your chest.

3. Slowly swing knees to your right side until they touch the floor, releasing left shoulder from the floor.

4. Repeat, swinging knees to left side.

5. Do this sequence 4 times.

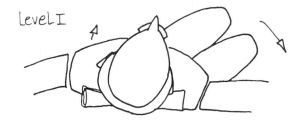

Level I

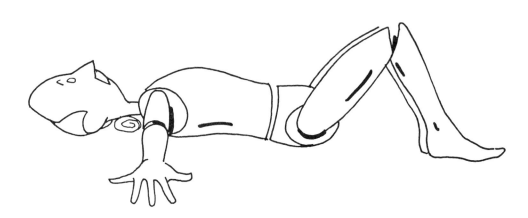

LEVEL III
ROLL OVERS:

1. Lie on your back, knees slightly bent, arms outstretched at shoulder level.

2. Lifting feet off the floor, bring your knees toward your chest.

3. Slowly swing knees to your right side until they touch the floor, releasing left shoulder from the floor.

4. Repeat, swinging knees to left side.

5. Do this sequence 6 times.

Remember:

- place towel under the nape of your neck for support

- if you have back problems, keep your feet on the floor when doing these exercises

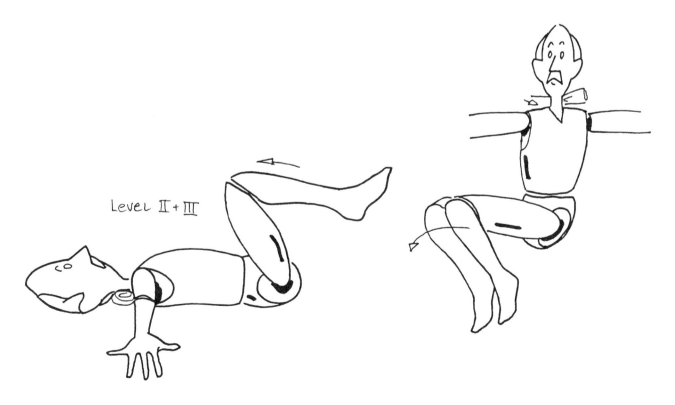

Level II + III

WARM-UP: LET'S LOOSEN UP!

**SESSION 3 - LEVEL I
LEG RAISES:**

1. Stand with left side toward the wall at arm's length. Place palm flat against the wall at shoulder height.

2. Slowly lift right leg to front, and lower.

3. Slowly lift right leg to side, and lower.

4. Slowly lift right leg to the back, and lower.

5. Do this sequence 4 times.

6. Turn around, place right hand on wall.

7. Repeat exercise with left leg.

**LEVEL II
LEG RAISES:**

1. Stand with left side toward the wall at arm's length. Place palm flat against the wall at shoulder height.

2. Slowly lift right leg to knee height at the front, bend knee bringing foot close to your body.

3. Return to starting position.

4. Repeat this movement, lifting and bending leg to the side, then to the back.

5. Do this sequence 4 times.

6. Turn around, place right hand on wall.

7. Repeat this exercise with left leg.

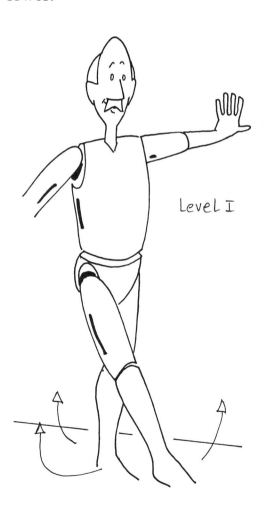

Level I

LEVEL III
LEG RAISES:

1. Stand with left side toward the wall at arm's length. Place palm flat against the wall at shoulder height.

2. Slowly lift right leg to knee height at the front, bend knee bringing foot close to your body.

3. Return to starting position.

4. Repeat this movement, lifting and bending leg to the side, then to the back.

5. Do this sequence 6 times.

6. Turn around, place opposite hand on wall.

7. Repeat this exercise with left leg.

Remember:

- do not arch back — especially when lifting leg behind you
- stand up straight

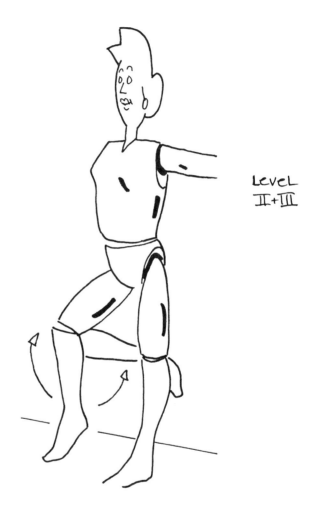

Level
II + III

WARM-UP: LET'S LOOSEN UP!

SESSION 3 - LEVEL I
TOES IN AND OUT:

1. Stand facing the wall at arm's length. Place palm flat against the wall at shoulder height, feet shoulder width apart.

2. Keeping heels on the floor, turn feet inward, describing a semicircle with your toes.

3. Return to starting position.

4. Do this sequence 4 times.

LEVEL II
TOES IN AND OUT:

1. Sit on the floor, back straight, knees bent toward your chest, feet flat on the floor, shoulder width apart.

2. Flex both feet so that toes are pointing toward the ceiling.

3. Keeping heels on the floor, turn feet inward trying to touch the inside of your feet to the floor.

4. Describing a semicircle, swing toes outward, trying to touch the outside of your feet to the floor.

5. Return to starting position.

6. Do this sequence 4 times.

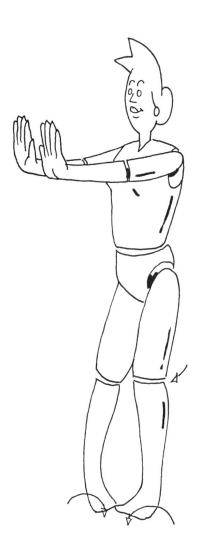

LEVEL III
TOES IN AND OUT:

1. Sit on the floor, back straight, knees bent toward your chest, feet flat on the floor, shoulder width apart.

2. Flex both feet so that toes are pointing toward the ceiling.

3. Keeping heels on the floor, turn feet inward trying to touch the inside of your feet to the floor.

4. Describing a semicircle, swing toes outward, trying to touch the outside of your feet to the floor.

5. Return to starting position.

6. Do this sequence 6 times.

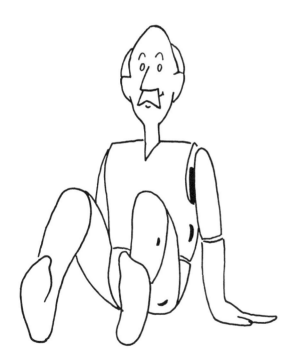

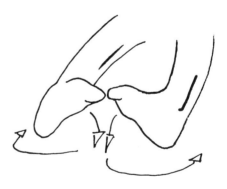

BODY OF THE CLASS: LET'S ENERGIZE!

SESSION 3 - LEVEL I

TOTAL TIME: 6 minutes

PUT ON SOME UPBEAT MUSIC

WHILE STANDING, DO THE FOLLOWING MOVEMENTS FOR 30 SECONDS EACH:

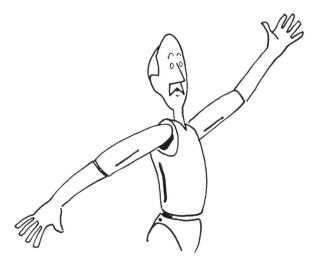

1. Walk on the spot.

2. March, lifting knees and swinging arms.

3. Continue marching, reach right arm then left arm toward the ceiling.
   ✱

4. Step side to side.

5. Kick right then left leg diagonally in front of you.

6. Continue this step, reach both arms toward the ceiling.

7. Lifting knees, touch right elbow to right knee, then left elbow to left knee.
   ✱

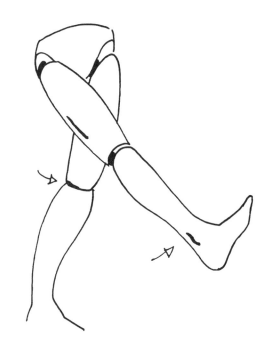

8. Point right foot in front on the floor. Repeat with left foot.

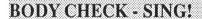
BODY CHECK - SING!

9. Continue pointing, cross arms in front and back.

10. Kick legs in front, swing arms above head.

11 . Walk slowly on the spot.

12 . Step side to side.

Stretch both arms above your head and breathe in deeply (3 times).

BODY CHECK - MONITOR HEART RATE!

LEVEL II

TOTAL TIME: 7 minutes

Do Level I and when you come to an * add a march with a hop for 30 seconds.

LEVEL III

TOTAL TIME: 9 minutes

Do Level I and when you come to an * add a march with a hop, swinging arms for 1 minute.

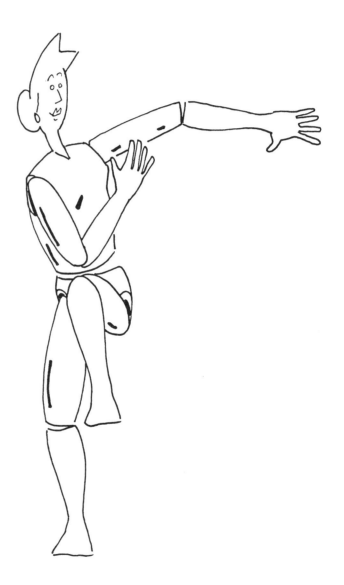

BODY OF THE CLASS: LET'S TONE UP!

SESSION 3 - LEVEL I
FIGURES OF 8: Sets: 2

Imagine that a large elastic band is around your wrists and is pulling your arms toward the ceiling — pull against this force!

1. Place arms in front of body at shoulder level, wrists crossed and hands clasped.

2. Slowly draw a figure 8 in front of your body moving from right side to left side, keeping elbows straight (remember the elastic band!).

3. Do this sequence 6 times.

4. Rest.

6. Complete the required number of sets.

LEVEL II
FIGURE OF 8: Sets: 2

With your weights around your wrists, do Level I .

LEVEL III
FIGURE OF 8: Sets: 2

With your weights around your wrists, do Level I .

Remember:

- do not arch back

- keep this movement slow and smooth

- do not forget to breathe

- keep knees slightly bent when doing this exercise

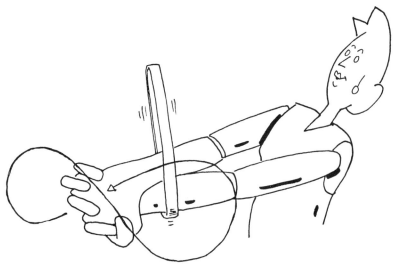

BODY OF THE CLASS: LET'S TONE UP!

| SESSION 3 - LEVEL I |
| RESISTANCE CURL: Sets: 2 |

1. Stretch right arm in front of your body, palm facing ceiling.

2. Place left arm on top of right arm, palms facing each other, clasp hands.

3. While breathing out, slowly bend arms toward the body, pressing left arm down (feel the resistance) (count 1,2,3).

4. Breathe in.

5. While breathing out, slowly stretch arms, pressing right arm up (feel the resistance) (count 1,2,3).

6. Do this sequence 6 times.

7. Rest.

8. Complete the required number of sets.

9. Repeat this exercise with right arm on top of left arm.

| LEVEL II |
| RESISTANCE CURL: Sets: 2 |

With your weights around your wrists, do Level I.

| LEVEL III |
| RESISTANCE CURL: Sets: 2 |

With your weights around your wrists, do Level I.

Remember:

- do not arch back
- keep this movement slow and smooth
- keep knees slightly bent when doing this exercise

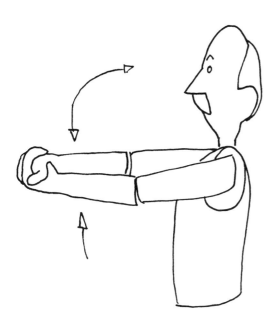

BODY OF THE CLASS: LET'S TONE UP!

SESSION 3 - LEVEL I
CURL UPS: Sets: 2

1. Lie on your back, bend knees toward chest, feet off the floor.

2. Place hands on thighs.

3. While breathing out, slowly raise head and both shoulder blades slightly off the floor (count 1,2,3).

4. While breathing in, slowly lower shoulders to the floor (count 1,2,3).

5. Do this sequence 3 times.

6. Rest.

7. Complete the required number of sets.

LEVEL II
CURL UPS: Sets: 2

1. Lie on your back, bend knees with feet flat on the floor.

2. Place hands on thighs.

3. While breathing out, slowly raise head and upper body slightly off the floor, (count 1,2,3).

4. While breathing in, slowly lower shoulders to the floor (count 1,2,3).

5. Do this sequence 3 times.

6. Rest.

7. Complete the required number of sets.

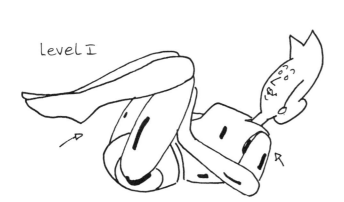

Level I

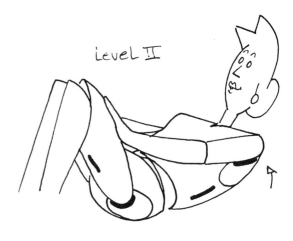

Level II

LEVEL III
CURL UPS: Sets: 2

1. Lie on your back, bend knees with feet flat on the floor.

2. Cross arms and place hands on shoulders.

3. While breathing out, slowly raise head and upper body off the floor, making sure that *only* your waist remains on the floor (count 1,2,3).

4. While breathing in, slowly lower shoulders to the floor (count 1,2,3).

5. Do this sequence 3 times.

6. Rest.

7. Complete the required number of sets.

Remember:
- make sure that shoulders touch the floor after each curl up
- raise *both* shoulder blades
- if you have difficulty keeping your feet on the floor, place weights around your ankles
- do not attempt to do a full sit up

Level III

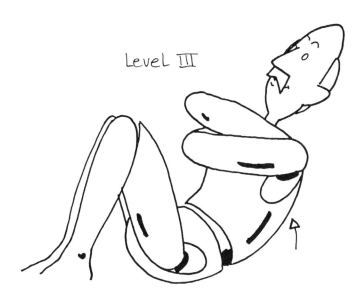

BODY OF THE CLASS: LET'S TONE UP!

SESSION 3 - LEVEL I
THE SQUEEZE: Sets: 2

1. Lie on your back, bend knees with feet flat on the floor and shoulder width apart.

2. Lift your hips so that your bottom is slightly off the floor.

3. Squeeze your bottom tightly (as if you are trying to hold something) (count 1,2,3).

4. Slowly lower your bottom to the floor.

5. Relax.

6. Do this sequence 3 times.

7. Rest.

8. Complete the required number of sets.

LEVEL II
THE SQUEEZE: Sets: 2

1. Lie on your back, bend knees with feet flat on the floor, knees and feet together.

2. Lift your hips so that your bottom is slightly off the floor.

3. Squeeze your bottom and inner thighs tightly (count 1,2,3).

4. Slowly lower your bottom to the floor.

5. Relax.

6. Do this sequence 3 times.

7. Rest.

8. Complete the required number of sets.

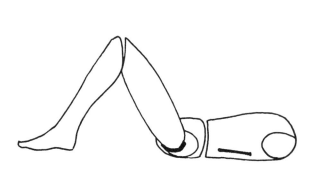

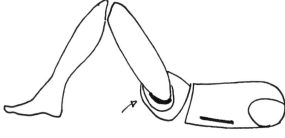

LEVEL III
THE SQUEEZE: Sets: 2

1. Lie on your back, bend knees with feet flat on the floor, knees and feet together.

2. Lift your hips so that your bottom is slightly off the floor.

3. Squeeze your bottom and inner thighs tightly.

4. Holding this squeeze, slowly sway hips to the right and then to the left.

5. Slowly lower your bottom to the floor.

6. Relax.

7. Do this sequence 3 times.

8. Rest.

9. Complete the required number of sets.

Remember:

- do not arch back
- keep this movement slow and smooth
- do not forget to breathe

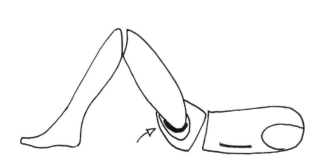
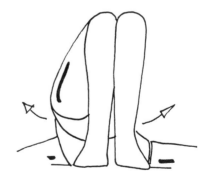

BODY OF THE CLASS: LET'S TONE UP!

SESSION 3 - LEVEL I
TIGHTEN AND LIFT: Sets: 2

1. Sit on the floor, back straight, right leg outstretched and left knee bent.

2. Place hands on floor behind you.

3. Straighten right leg and flex your foot while tightening the thigh muscle.

4. Lift right leg so that heel is approximately 1 foot off the floor (count 1,2,3).

5. Slowly lower leg to the floor (count 1,2,3).

6. Repeat this exercise with the left leg.

7. Do this sequence 3 times.

8. Rest.

9. Complete the required number of sets.

LEVEL II
TIGHTEN AND LIFT: Sets: 2

With your weights around your ankles, do Level I.

LEVEL II
TIGHTEN AND LIFT: Sets: 2

With your weights around your ankles, do Level I.

Remember:

- keep this movement slow and smooth

- do not forget to breathe

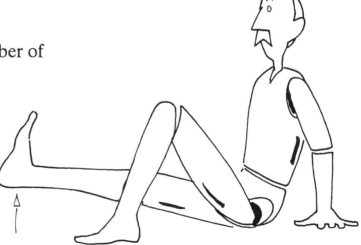

BODY OF THE CLASS: LET'S TONE UP!

SESSION 3 - LEVEL I
CIRCLES IN THE AIR: Sets: 2

1. Lie on your left side, head resting on left arm, legs in straight line with your upper body.

2. Point right foot and slowly lift right leg as high as possible, hips facing forward.

3. With right leg in the air, describe 3 large circles to the front.

4. Lower right leg to rest on left leg.

5. Lift right leg as high as possible, pointing toes, hips facing forward.

6. With right leg in the air, describe 3 large circles to the back.

7. Lower leg.

8. Rest.

9. Complete the required number of sets.

10. Turn over so that you are lying on your right side.

11. Repeat these exercises with left leg.

LEVEL II
CIRCLES IN THE AIR: Sets: 2

With your weights around your ankles, do Level I.

LEVEL III
CIRCLES IN THE AIR: Sets: 2

With your weights around your ankles, do Level I.

Remember:

- do not arch back
- keep upper body still when lifting leg
- use hand on floor in front of you for support
- keep this movement slow and smooth
- do not forget to breathe

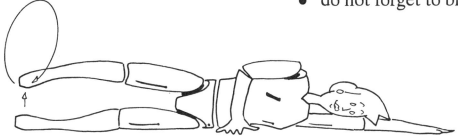

COOL-DOWN: LET'S STRETCH!

SESSION 3 - LEVEL I
HOLDING STRETCH:

1. Lift your left arm toward the ceiling, fingers pointing upward.

2. Bend upper body to the right, tilt head toward right shoulder.

3. Stretch and hold this position for 4 seconds.

4. Return to **BASIC POSITION.**

5. Repeat this exercise to the left side.

6. Do this sequence 3 times.

LEVEL II
HOLDING STRETCH:

1. Put your right hand on the small of your back.

2. Lift your left arm toward the ceiling, fingers pointing upward.

3. Bend upper body to the right, tilt head toward right shoulder.

4. Stretch and hold this position for 4 seconds.

5. Return to **BASIC POSITION**.

6. Repeat this exercise to the left side.

7. Do this sequence 4 times.

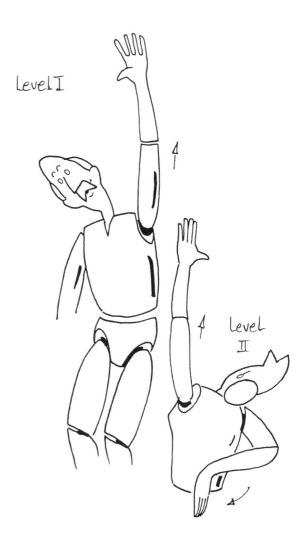

Level I

Level II

LEVEL III
HOLDING STRETCH:

1. Lift arms toward the ceiling, grab your left wrist with your right hand.

2. Bend your upper body to the right side while pulling on your wrist, tilt head toward right shoulder.

3. Stretch and hold this position for 5 seconds.

4. Return to **BASIC POSITION**.

5. Repeat this exercise with left hand holding right wrist and bending to the left.

6. Do this sequence 4 times.

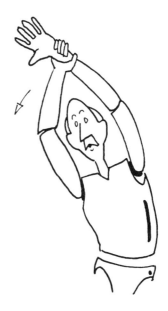

Remember:

- do not arch back

- keep knees slightly bent when doing this exercise

- do this exercise slowly

- always bend directly to the side, not forward or backward

- keep hips facing forward

- this exercise can be done while sitting on a chair or with your back against the wall

COOL-DOWN: LET'S STRETCH!

SESSION 3 - LEVEL I
REACH BACKS:

1. Cross right arm in front of your body and place right hand on left shoulder, left hand on hip.

2. Move right hand as far down your back as possible.

3. Reach and hold this position for 4 seconds.

4. Return to **BASIC POSITION**.

5. Keeping left hand on hip, place right hand on lower back and reach up your back as far as possible.

6. Reach and hold this position for 4 seconds.

7. Return to **BASIC POSITION**.

8. Repeat this exercise with left arm.

9. Do this sequence 3 times.

LEVEL II
REACH BACKS:

1. Cross right arm in front of body and place right hand on left shoulder.

2. Move right hand as far down your back as possible.

3. With left hand on right elbow, slowly and gently push elbow so that right hand moves further down your back.

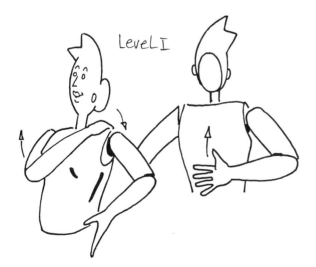

Level I

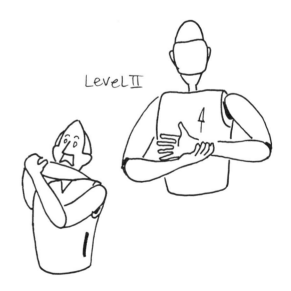

Level II

4. Hold this position for 4 seconds.

5. Return to **BASIC POSITION**.

6. Place right hand on lower back and reach up as far as possible.

7. With left hand behind your back, slowly and gently push right hand further up your back.

8. Hold this position for 4 seconds.

9. Return to **BASIC POSITION**.

10. Repeat this exercise with left arm.

11. Do this sequence 4 times.

LEVEL III
REACH BACKS:

---

1. Put your right hand on the small of your back.

2. Put your left hand on your left shoulder.

3. Slowly move your right hand up and slide your left hand down, trying to touch your fingers at the back.

4. Reach and hold this position for 5 seconds.

5. Return to **BASIC POSITION**.

6. Repeat this exercise with left hand on top.

7. Do this sequence 4 times.

If you find this exercise too difficult, place a towel in the hand on your shoulder and walk both hands toward each other along the towel.

Remember:
- do not arch back
- keep knees slightly bent when doing this exercise
- do this exercise slowly

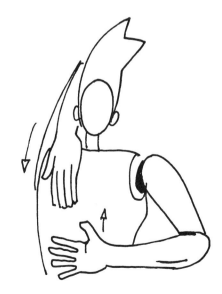

COOL-DOWN: LET'S STRETCH!

SESSION 3 - LEVEL I
THIGH STRETCHES:

1. Stand with left side toward the wall at arm's length. Place palm flat against the wall at shoulder height.

2. Lift right leg to the front toward the ceiling.

3. Flex foot with toes pointing toward the ceiling (tighten the muscles in your thigh).

4. Hold this position for 4 seconds.

5. Return to starting position.

6. Keeping your knees together, bend your right leg backward, flex your foot and try to touch your bottom with your heel.

7. Hold this position for 4 seconds.

8. Do this sequence 3 times.

9. Turn around and repeat this exercise on the other side.

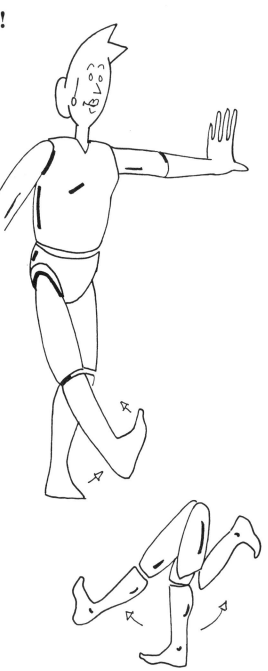

LEVEL II
THIGH STRETCHES:

1. Stand with left side toward the wall at arm's length. Place palm flat against the wall at shoulder height.

2. Lift right leg to the front toward the ceiling.

3. Flex foot with toes pointing toward the ceiling (tighten the muscles in your thigh).

4. Hold this position for 4 seconds.

5. Return to starting position.

6. Keeping your knees together, bend your right leg backward, flex your foot and try to touch your bottom with your heel.

7. Hold this position for 4 seconds.

8. Do this sequence 4 times.

9. Turn around and repeat this exercise on the other side.

LEVEL III
THIGH STRETCHES:

1. Stand with left side toward the wall at arm's length. Place palm flat against the wall at shoulder height.

2. Lift right leg to the front toward the ceiling.

3. Flex foot with toes pointing toward the ceiling (tighten the muscles in your thigh).

4. Hold this position for 5 seconds.

5. Return to starting position.

6. Keeping your knees together, bend your right leg backward, flex your foot and try to touch your bottom with your heel.

7. Hold this position for 5 seconds.

8. Do this sequence 4 times.

9. Turn around and repeat this exercise on the other side.

Remember:
- keep supporting knee bent
- do this exercise slowly

COOL-DOWN: LET'S STRETCH!

SESSION 3 - LEVEL I
SPINAL TWIST:

1. Lie on your back, knees slightly bent, arms out to the side.

2. Bend right knee so that right foot is beside left knee.

3. Cross right knee over left leg toward the floor on your left side, releasing right shoulder from the floor.

4. Stretch and hold this position for 4 seconds.

5. Return to starting position.

6. Repeat this exercise with left leg.

7. Do this sequence 3 times.

LEVEL II
SPINAL TWIST:

1. Lie on your back, knees slightly bent, arms out to the side.

2. Bend right knee so that right foot is beside left knee.

3. Cross right knee over left leg toward the floor on your left side.

4. Swing arms to right side (look at your hands).

5. Hold this position for 4 seconds.

6. Return to starting position.

7. Repeat this exercise with left leg.

8. Do this sequence 4 times.

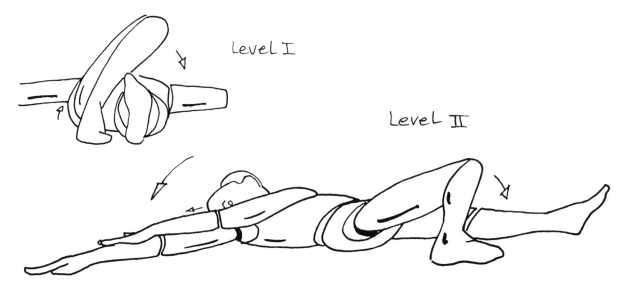

Level I

Level II

LEVEL III
SPINAL TWISTS:

1. Lie on your back, knees slightly bent, arms out to the side.

2. Bend right knee so that right foot is beside left knee.

3. Cross right knee over left leg toward the floor on your left side, releasing right shoulder from the floor.

4. Place left hand on right knee and gently and slowly press knee toward the floor.

5. Hold this position for 5 seconds.

6. Return to starting position.

7. Repeat this exercise with left leg.

8. Do this sequence 4 times.

Remember:
- do not force these positions
- do this exercise slowly and smoothly

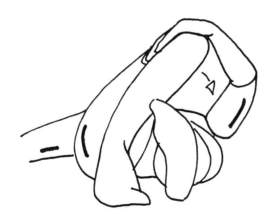

COOL-DOWN: LET'S RELAX!

SESSION 3 - LEVEL I

READ THE COMPLETE
RELAXATION EXERCISE
BEFORE YOU BEGIN.

TOTAL TIME: 4 minutes

1. Turn on soft background music.

2. Lie on your back and cover yourself with a warm blanket.

3. Lift one leg at a time a few inches off the floor and lower it, completely relaxed.

4. Lift arms slightly off the floor and lower them, completely relaxed.

5. Shrug shoulders, and relax.

6. Arch your back slightly and relax.

7. Lift your head slightly and relax.

8. Wrinkle your face and relax.

9. Breathe slowly until your body is completely relaxed.

10. Let this relaxed feeling flow through your body — ENJOY.

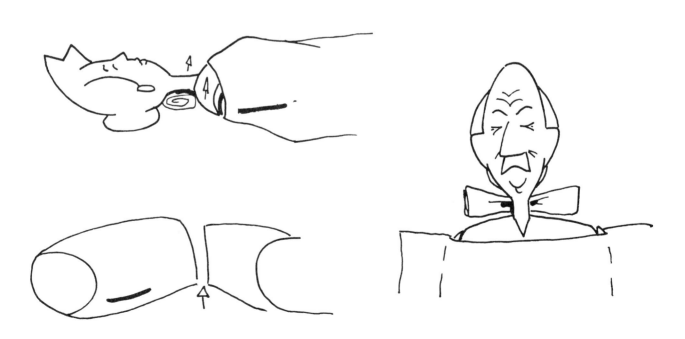

LEVEL II

Do Level I.

LEVEL III

Do Level I.

Remember:

- if possible, turn off some of the lights where you will be relaxing

- relax in a quiet area

- keep your breathing slow and rhythmic

- close your eyes when relaxing

- if you have a sleeping bag, use it rather than a blanket — it is excellent for these exercises

- be aware of the difference in your muscles when they are tensed or relaxed

- use a towel or a small pillow at the nape of your neck for support

- if you have lower back problems support your legs on the seat of a chair

LET'S GET FIT - SESSION 4

WARM-UP: LET'S BEGIN!

SESSION 4 - LEVEL I

TOTAL TIME: 4 minutes

PUT ON SOME LIVELY MUSIC.

1. Kick right leg in front, then left leg, at a slow relaxed pace for 30 seconds.

2. Continue kicking and do the following movements for 30 seconds each:

a) swing hips from side to side

b) extend right arm above head, then left arm

c) flex feet as you kick

d) clap hands front and back

e) swing arms from side to side above head

f) kick right then left leg to the side

g) gradually, step more slowly

3. Stretch both arms above your head and breathe in deeply (3 times).

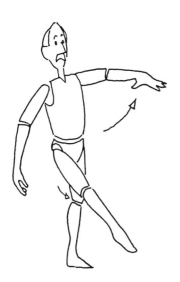

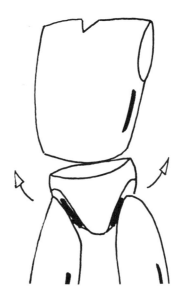

LEVEL II
Do Level I.

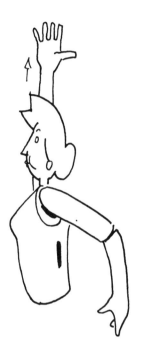

LEVEL III
Do Level I.

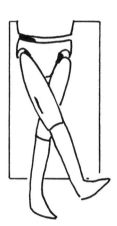

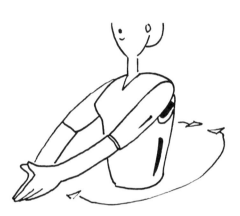

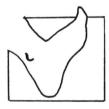

WARM-UP: LET'S LOOSEN UP!

SESSION 4 - LEVEL I
HEAD ROLLS:

1. Lean head to the right, bringing your ear toward your shoulder.

2. In a smooth, continuous motion, roll your head toward the front and describe a semicircle moving from your right shoulder to your left shoulder.

3. Repeat this exercise in the opposite direction.

4. Do this sequence 4 times.

LEVEL II
HEAD ROLLS:

1. Place your arms down along the sides of your body; press heels of hands toward the floor. Keep this tension in your arms and...

2. Lean head to the right, bringing your ear toward your shoulder. Press heel of left hand further toward the floor.

3. In a smooth, continuous motion, roll your head toward the front moving from your right shoulder to your left shoulder. Press heel of right hand further toward the floor.

4. Repeat this exercise in the opposite direction.

5. Do this sequence 4 times.

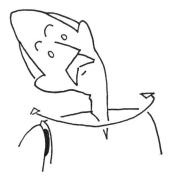

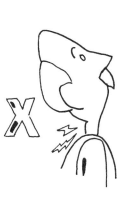

LEVEL III
HEAD ROLLS:

1. Place your arms down along the sides of your body; press heels of hands toward the floor. Keep this tension in your arms and...

2. Lean head to the right, bringing your ear toward your shoulder. Press heel of left hand further toward the floor.

3. In a smooth, continuous motion, roll your head toward the front moving from your right shoulder to your left shoulder. Press heel of right hand further toward the floor.

4. Repeat this exercise in the opposite direction.

5. Do this sequence 6 times.

Remember:

- do not tilt head backward
- keep shoulders still

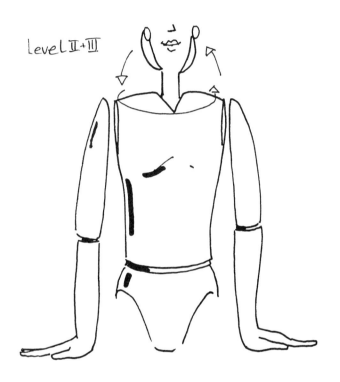

Level II + III

WARM-UP: LET'S LOOSEN UP!

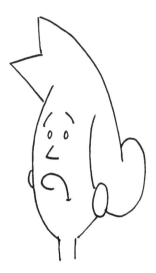

SESSION 4 - LEVEL I
POUTS:

1. Exaggerate a pout.

2. Pull your chin downward, opening your mouth.

3. Relax.

4. Do this sequence 4 times.

LEVEL II
POUTS:

1. Exaggerate a pout.

2. Pull your chin downward, opening your mouth widely; try to touch your tongue to the roof of your mouth.

3. Relax.

4. Do this sequence 4 times.

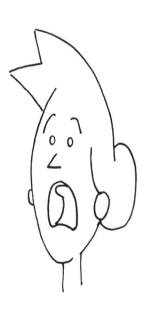

LEVEL III
POUTS:

1. Exaggerate a pout.

2. Pull your chin downward, opening your mouth widely, try to touch your tongue to the roof of your mouth.

3. Relax.

4. Do this sequence 6 times.

WARM-UP: LET'S LOOSEN UP!

SESSION 4 - LEVEL I
CRAWLS:

1. Place your hands on your shoulders, elbows up.

2. Try to touch your elbows together in front of your body.

3. In a circular motion, bring elbows up to the side, down, and back to the front.

4. Do this sequence 4 times.

5. Repeat in the opposite direction.

LEVEL II
CRAWLS:

1. Hold your arms out to the side at shoulder height, elbows bent with hands toward the ceiling. Keeping arms at this level...

2. Try to touch your elbows together in front of your body.

3. In a circular motion, bring elbows up to the side, down, and back to the front.

4. Do this sequence 4 times.

5. Repeat in the opposite direction.

LEVEL III
CRAWLS:

1. Hold your arms out to the side at shoulder height, elbows bent with hands toward the ceiling. Keeping arms at this level..

2. Try to touch your elbows together in front of your body.

3. In a circular motion, bring elbows up to the side, down, and back to the front.

4. Do this sequence 6 times.

5. Repeat in the opposite direction.

Remember:

- keep a slow, smooth rhythm

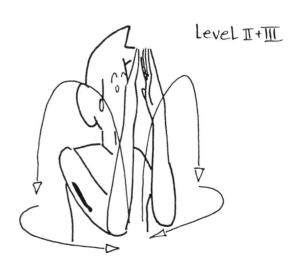

Level II+III

WARM-UP: LET'S LOOSEN UP!

SESSION 4 - LEVEL I
WRIST FLEXES:

1. With palms facing ceiling, make a fist with your right hand.

2. Hold right forearm with left hand.

3. Bend fist downward as far as possible.

4. Bend fist upward as far as possible.

5. Bend fist side to side.

6. Do this sequence 4 times.

7. Repeat with other hand.

LEVEL II
WRIST FLEXES:

1. With palms facing ceiling, holding your right forearm with your left hand, extend the fingers of your right hand.

2. Bend fingers downward as far as possible.

3. Bend fingers upward as far as possible.

4. Bend fingers side to side as far as possible.

5. Do this sequence 4 times.

6. Repeat with other hand.

LEVEL III
WRIST FLEXES:

1. With palms facing ceiling, holding your right forearm with your left hand, extend the fingers of your right hand.

2. Bend fingers downward as far as possible.

3. Bend fingers upward as far as possible.

4. Bend fingers side to side as far as possible.

5. Do this sequence 6 times.

6. Repeat with other hand.

Remember:

- try to keep forearms still, the action is in the wrist

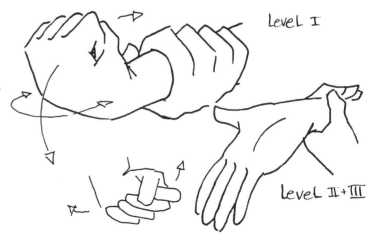

Level I

Level II + III

WARM-UP: LET'S LOOSEN UP!

SESSION 4 - LEVEL I
FIST CLENCHES:

1. Spread the fingers of both hands as far apart as possible.

2. Make a fist and open it, spreading fingers wide.

3. Do this sequence 4 times.

LEVEL II
FIST CLENCHES:

1. Spread the fingers of both hands as far apart as possible.

2. Make fists.

3. Squeeze and tighten these fists as much as possible.

4. Spread fingers of your hands as far apart as possible.

5. Do this sequence 4 times.

LEVEL III
FIST CLENCHES:

1. Spread the fingers of both hands as far apart as possible.

2. Make fists.

3. Squeeze and tighten these fists as much as possible.

4. Spread fingers of your hands as far apart as possible.

5. Do this sequence 6 times.

Remember:
- keep movements slow and smooth
- do not force this movement

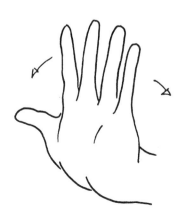 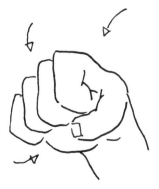 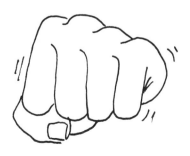

WARM-UP: LET'S LOOSEN UP!

SESSION 4 - LEVEL I
WAIST TWISTS:

1. Place left hand on hip and raise right arm above head.

2. Turn to the left to look behind you, twisting your upper body.

3. Return to starting position.

4. Repeat on the other side.

5. Do this sequence 4 times.

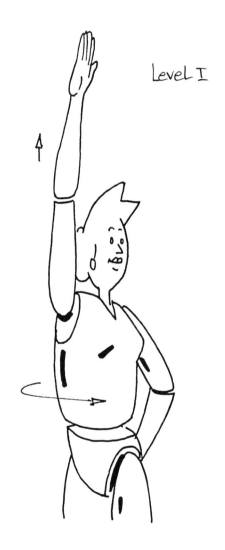

Level I

LEVEL II
WAIST TWISTS:

1. Stand approximately 1 foot away from the wall, back toward the wall.

2. Place left hand on hip and raise right arm above head.

3. Twisting your upper body to the left, turn to look behind you, trying to place your right hand on the wall.

4. Return to starting position.

5. Repeat this exercise on the other side.

6. Do this sequence 4 times.

LEVEL III
WAIST TWISTS:

1. Stand approximately 1 foot away from the wall, back toward the wall.

2. Place left hand on hip and raise right arm above head.

3. Twisting your upper body to the left, turn to look behind you, trying to place your right hand on the wall.

4. Return to starting position.

5. Repeat this exercise on the other side.

6. Do this sequence 6 times.

Remember:

- do not arch back

- do not lock knees

- you can perform this exercise sitting down

- keep this movement slow and smooth

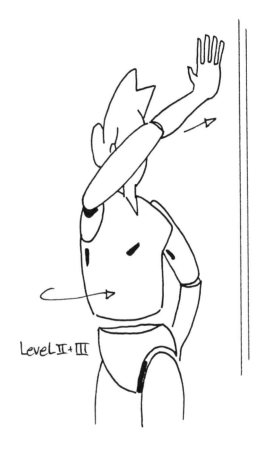

Level II + III

WARM-UP: LET'S LOOSEN UP!

SESSION 4 - LEVEL I
LEG SWINGS:

1. Stand with left side toward the wall at arm's length. Place palm flat against the wall at shoulder height.

2. Slowly swing right leg forward and backward, bringing it to knee height.

3. Do this sequence 4 times.

4. Turn around, place opposite hand on the wall.

5. Repeat exercise with left leg.

LEVEL II
LEG SWINGS:

1. Stand with left side toward the wall at arm's length. Place palm flat against the wall at shoulder height.

2. Slowly swing right leg forward and backward, bringing it as high as possible.

3. Do this sequence 4 times.

4. Turn around, place opposite hand on the wall.

5. Repeat exercise with left leg.

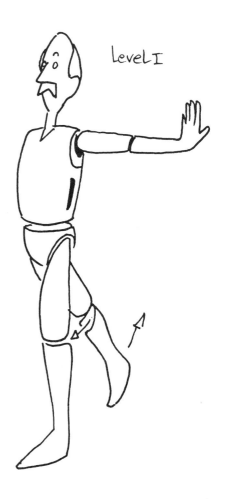

Level I

LEVEL III
LEG SWINGS:

1. Stand with left side toward the wall at arm's length. Place palm flat against the wall at shoulder height.

2. Slowly swing right leg forward and backward, bringing it as high as possible.

3. Do this sequence 6 times.

4. Turn around, place opposite hand on the wall.

5. Repeat exercise with left leg.

Remember:

- do not arch your back
- keep this movement slow and smooth

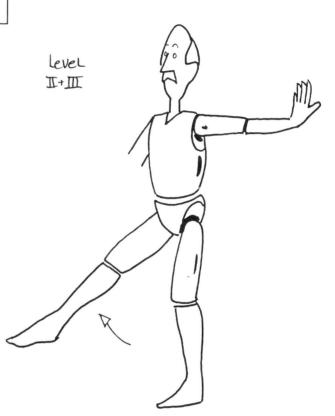

Level
II + III

WARM-UP: LET'S LOOSEN UP!

SESSION 4 - LEVEL I
HEEL CIRCLES:

1. Stand with left side toward the wall at arm's length. Place palm flat against the wall at shoulder height.

2. Bend right knee toward your chest, lifting toes off the floor.

3. Flex right foot, toes pointing toward the ceiling.

4. Point right foot, toes pointing toward the floor.

5. Turn foot to the right, then the left.

6. Do this sequence 4 times.

7. Turn around, place opposite hand on wall.

8. Repeat exercise with left foot.

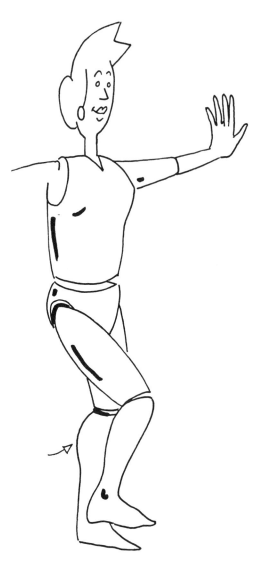

Level I

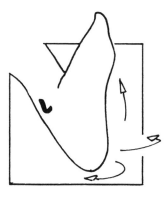 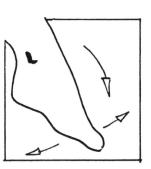

LEVEL II HEEL CIRCLES:	LEVEL III HEEL CIRCLES:

1. Stand with left side toward the wall at arm's length. Place palm flat against the wall at shoulder height.

2. Bend right knee and place tip of big toe on the floor.

3. Describe 4 circles with your heel, keeping big toe on the floor.

4. Repeat exercise reversing the direction of the circles.

5. Turn around, place opposite hand on wall.

6. Repeat exercise with left foot.

1. Stand with left side toward the wall at arm's length. Place palm flat against the wall at shoulder height.

2. Bend right knee and place tip of big toe on the floor.

3. Describe 6 circles with your heel, keeping big toe on the floor.

4. Repeat exercise reversing the direction of the circles.

5. Turn around, place opposite hand on wall.

6. Repeat exercise with left foot.

Level II + III

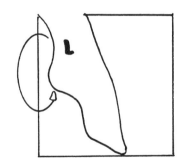

BODY OF THE CLASS: LET'S ENERGIZE!

SESSION 4 - LEVEL I

TOTAL TIME: 6 minutes

PUT ON SOME UPBEAT MUSIC

WHILE STANDING, DO THE FOLLOWING MOVEMENTS FOR 30 SECONDS EACH:

1. Walk on the spot.

2. March, lifting knees and swinging arms.

3. While lifting knees, clap hands under thigh.

4. While lifting knees, touch opposite elbow to knee.

5. Step side to side.

BODY CHECK - SING!

6. Continue stepping side to side, swinging arms up and down in front of body.

7. Continue stepping side to side, swinging arms side to side above head.

8. March .

BODY CHECK - SING!

9. Continue marching, reaching right arm then left arm toward the ceiling.

10. Continue marching, swinging arms.

11. Continue marching, crossing arms above head.

12. March slowly.

13. Walk on the spot.

Stretch both arms above your head and breathe in deeply (4 times).

BODY CHECK - MONITOR HEART RATE!

LEVEL II

TOTAL TIME: 8 minutes

Do Level I and when you come to an
* add a march with a hop for 30
seconds.

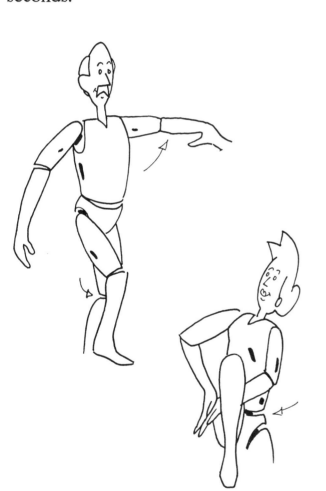

LEVEL III

TOTAL TIME: 9 minutes

Do Level I and when you come to an
* add a march with a hop, swinging
arms for 1 minute.

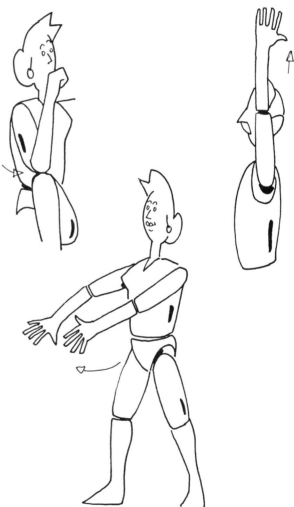

BODY OF THE CLASS: LET'S TONE UP!

SESSION 4 - LEVEL I
ROUND ABOUTS: Sets: 3

Imagine that a large elastic band is around your wrists and is pulling your arms toward the ceiling — pull against this force!

1. Stretch arms out to the side at shoulder level, fingers pointing toward the ceiling.

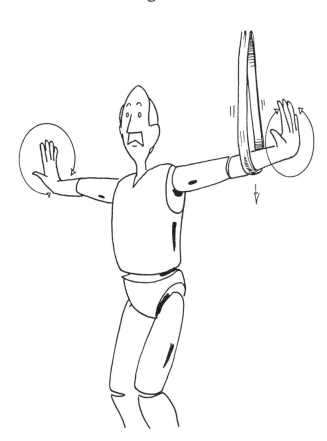

2. Describe 7 small circles with your arms going forward (remember the elastic band!).

3. Repeat this exercise circling backward (remember the elastic band!).

4. Rest.

5. Complete the required number of sets.

LEVEL II
ROUND ABOUTS: Sets: 3

With your weights around your wrists, do Level I.

LEVEL III
ROUND ABOUTS: Sets: 3

With your weights around your wrists, do Level I.

Remember:

- do not arch back
- keep this movement slow and smooth
- do not forget to breathe
- keep knees slightly bent when doing this exercise

BODY OF THE CLASS: LET'S TONE UP!

SESSION 4 - LEVEL I
CURL AND PRESS: Sets: 3

1. Place arms straight out in front of you at shoulder level, palms up, make tight fists and...

2. While breathing out, bring fists to touch shoulders (as if to lift a heavy object) (count 1,2,3).

3. While breathing in, turn fists to face the front.

4. While breathing out, press fists toward the ceiling (as if to lift a heavy object) (count 1,2,3).

5. Return to starting position.

6. Do this sequence 7 times.

7. Rest.

8. Complete the required number of sets.

LEVEL II
CURL AND PRESS: Sets: 3

With your weights around your wrists, do Level I.

LEVEL III
CURL AND PRESS: Sets: 3

With your weights around your wrists, do Level I.

Remember:

- keep arms shoulder width apart
- keep this movement slow and smooth
- keep knees slightly bent when doing this exercise

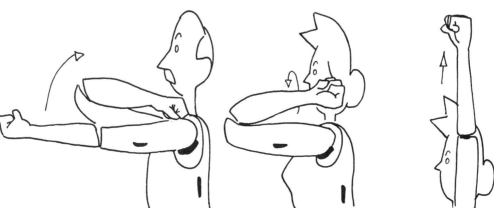

BODY OF THE CLASS: LET'S TONE UP!

| SESSION 4 - LEVEL I
UP AND OVERS: Sets: 3 | LEVEL II
UP AND OVERS: Sets: 3 |

1. Lie on your back, bend knees toward chest, feet off the floor.

2. Place hands on thighs.

3. While breathing out, slowly raise head and both shoulder blades slightly off the floor and touch the outside of your right knee with your left hand (count 1,2,3).

4. While breathing in, slowly lower shoulders to the floor (count 1,2,3).

5. Repeat this exercise on the other side.

6. Do this sequence 3 times.

7. Rest.

8. Complete the required number of sets.

1. Lie on your back, bend knees keep your feet flat on the floor.

2. Place hands on thighs .

3. While breathing out, slowly raise head and both shoulder blades slightly off the floor. Try to touch the outside of your right knee with your left hand (count 1,2,3).

4. While breathing in, slowly lower shoulders to the floor (count 1,2,3).

5. Repeat this exercise on the other side.

6. Do this sequence 3 times.

7. Rest.

8. Complete the required number of sets.

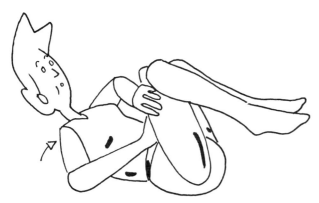

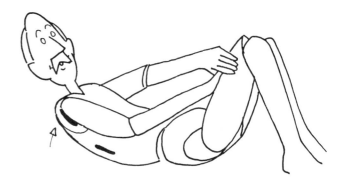

LEVEL III
UP AND OVERS: Sets: 3

1. Lie on your back, bend your knees with feet flat on the floor.

2. Cross arms and place hands on shoulders.

3. While breathing out, slowly raise head and upper body off the floor making sure that *only* your waist remains on the floor (count 1,2,3).

4. Try to touch your right knee with your left elbow.

5. While breathing in, slowly lower shoulders to the floor (count 1,2,3).

6. Repeat this exercise on the other side.

7. Do this sequence 3 times.

8. Rest.

9. Complete the required number of sets.

Remember:

- if you have difficulty keeping your feet on the floor, place weights around your ankles

- make sure that shoulders touch the floor after each curl up

- raise *both* shoulder blades

- do not attempt to do a full sit up

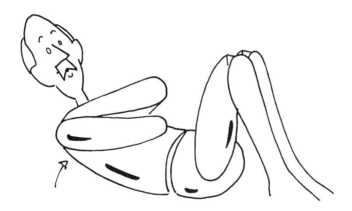

BODY OF THE CLASS: LET'S TONE UP!

SESSION 4 - LEVEL I
KNEE DROP SQUEEZE: Sets: 3

1. Lie on your back, bend knees with feet flat on the floor and shoulder width apart.

2. Keeping feet still, bring knees together.

3. Lift your hips so that your bottom is slightly off the floor.

4. Squeeze your bottom tightly (as if you are trying to hold something) (count 1,2,3).

5. Slowly lower your bottom to the floor.

6. Relax.

7. Do this sequence 3 times.

8. Rest.

9. Complete the required number of sets.

LEVEL II
KNEE DROP SQUEEZE: Sets: 3

1. Lie on your back, bend knees with feet flat on the floor and shoulder width apart.

2. Keeping feet still, bring knees together.

3. Lift your hips so that your bottom is slightly off the floor.

4. Squeeze your bottom tightly (as if you are trying to hold something) (count 1,2,3).

5. Slowly lower your bottom *almost* to the floor.

6. Raise hips once again.

7. Do this sequence 3 times.

8. Rest.

9. Complete the required number of sets.

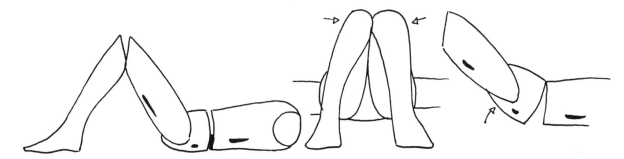

LEVEL III
KNEE DROP SQUEEZE: Sets: 3

1. Lie on your back, bend knees with feet flat on the floor and shoulder width apart.

2. Keeping feet still, bring knees together.

3. Lift your hips so that your bottom is slightly off the floor.

4. Squeeze your bottom tightly (as if you are trying to hold something) (count 1,2,3).

5. Keeping feet still, open your knees as far as possible.

6. Keeping feet still, close your knees.

7. Slowly lower your bottom *almost* to the floor.

8. Raise hips once again.

9. Do this sequence 3 times.

10 Rest.

11. Complete the required number of sets.

Remember:
- do not arch back
- keep this movement slow and smooth
- do not forget to breathe

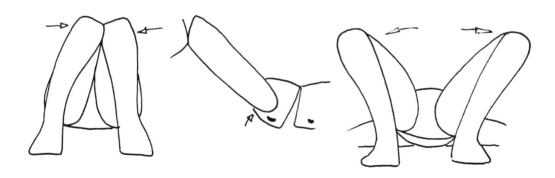

BODY OF THE CLASS: LET'S TONE UP!

SESSION 4 - LEVEL I
TIGHTEN AND SWING: Sets: 3

1. Sit on the floor, back straight, right leg outstretched and left knee bent.

2. Place hands on floor behind you.

3. Flex your right foot so that toes are pointing toward the ceiling (tighten your thigh muscles).

4. Keeping muscles tightened, slowly lift right leg until it is approximately 1 foot off the floor.

5. *Slowly* swing it to your right side.

6. Slowly lower leg to the floor.

7. Lifting right leg off the floor, bring it back to the centre.

8. Slowly lower leg to the floor.

9. Repeat this exercise with your left leg.

10. Do this sequence 3 times.

11. Rest.

12. Complete the required number of sets.

LEVEL II
TIGHTEN AND SWING: Sets: 3

With your weights around your ankles, do Level I.

LEVEL III
TIGHTEN AND SWING: Sets: 3

With your weights around your ankles, do Level I.

Remember:

- keep this movement slow and smooth

- do not forget to breathe

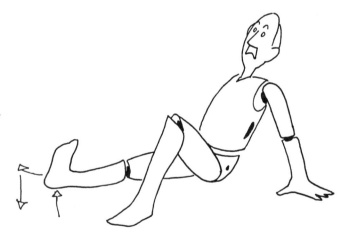

BODY OF THE CLASS: LET'S TONE UP!

SESSION 4 - LEVEL I
SIDE & FRONT LEG LIFTS: Sets: 3

1. Lie on your left side, head resting on left arm, legs in straight line with your upper body.

2. With toes pointed, lift your right leg as high as possible, keeping hips facing forward.

3. Slowly bring your right foot forward and touch the floor with your right foot.

4. Raise your right leg in front, return it to the side and lower it to rest on left leg.

5. Do this sequence 3 times.

6. Rest.

7. Complete the required number of sets.

8. Turn over so that you lie on your right side.

9. Repeat this exercise with left leg.

LEVEL II
SIDE & FRONT LEG LIFTS: Sets: 3

With your weights around your ankles, do Level I.

LEVEL III
SIDE & FRONT LEG LIFTS: Sets: 3

With your weights around your ankles, do Level I.

Remember:

- do not arch back
- keep upper body still when lifting leg
- use hand on floor in front of you for support
- keep this movement slow and smooth
- do not forget to breathe

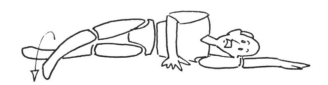

COOL-DOWN: LET'S STRETCH!

SESSION 4 - LEVEL I
SIDE PULLS:

1. Reach right hand over your head, bend your elbow and touch your left ear.

2. Stretch left arm toward the ceiling.

3. Keeping arms in these positions, bend upper body to the right.

4. Let right elbow become heavy, pulling your upper body down.

5. Stretch and hold this position for 4 seconds.

6. Return to **BASIC POSITION**.

7. Repeat this exercise to left side.

8. Do this sequence 4 times.

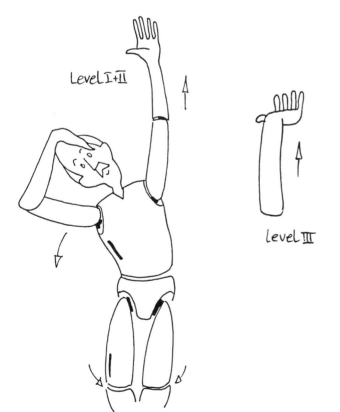

Level I+II

Level III

LEVEL II
SIDE PULLS:

1. Reach your right hand over your head, bend your elbow and touch your left ear.

2. Stretch left arm toward the ceiling.

3. Keeping arms in these positions, bend upper body to the right.

4. Let right elbow become heavy, pulling the upper body down.

5. Stretch and hold this position for 4 seconds.

6. Return to **BASIC POSITION**.

7. Repeat this exercise to left side.

8. Do this sequence 5 times.

LEVEL III
SIDE PULLS:

1. Reach your right hand over your head, bend your elbow and touch your left ear.

2. Stretch left arm toward the ceiling, wrist flexed, palm facing ceiling.

3. Keeping arms in these positions, bend upper body to the right.

4. Let right elbow become heavy, pulling the upper body down.

5. Stretch and hold this position for 5 seconds.

6. Return to **BASIC POSITION**.

7. Repeat this exercise to left side.

8. Do this sequence 5 times.

Remember:
- do not arch back
- keep knees slightly bent when doing this exercise
- do this exercise slowly
- always bend directly to the side, not forward or backward
- keep hips facing forward
- this exercise can be done while sitting on a chair or with your back against the wall

COOL-DOWN: LET'S STRETCH

SESSION 4 - LEVEL I
CHEST AND SHOULDER STRETCH:

1. Place right hand on the small of your back.

2. Grab fingertips of right hand with left hand and gently and slowly pull right arm to the left.

3. Hold this position for 4 seconds.

4. Return to **BASIC POSITION**.

5. Place right arm in front of body at shoulder level.

6. Grab fingertips of right hand with left hand and gently and slowly pull right arm to the left.

7. Hold this position for 4 seconds.

8. Do this sequence 4 times.

9. Repeat this exercise with your other arm.

Level I

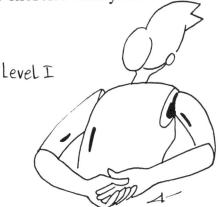

LEVEL II
CHEST AND SHOULDER STRETCH:

1. Place right hand on the small of your back.

2. Grab right wrist with left hand and gently and slowly pull right arm to the left.

3. Pull up gently.

4. Hold this position for 4 seconds.

5. Return to **BASIC POSITION**.

6. Place right arm in front of body at shoulder level.

7. Grab right wrist with left hand and gently and slowly pull right arm to the left.

8. Pull up gently.

9. Hold this position for 4 seconds.

10. Do this sequence 5 times.

11. Repeat this exercise with your other arm.

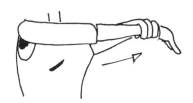

LEVEL III
CHEST AND SHOULDER STRETCH:

1. Place right hand on the small of your back.

2. Grab right arm with left hand and gently and slowly pull right arm to the left.

3. Pull up gently.

4. Hold this position for 5 seconds.

5. Return to **BASIC POSITION**.

6. Place right arm in front of body at shoulder level.

7. Grab right elbow with left hand and gently and slowly pull right arm to the left.

8. Pull up gently.

9. Hold this position for 5 seconds.

10. Do this sequence 5 times.

11. Repeat this exercise with your other arm.

Remember:

- do not arch back
- keep knees slightly bent when doing this exercise
- do this exercise slowly

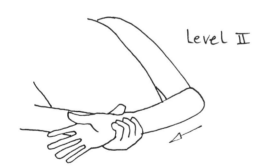

Level II

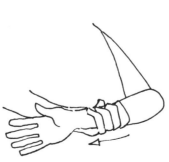

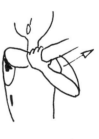

Level III

COOL-DOWN: LET'S STRETCH

SESSION 4 - LEVEL I
CALF STRETCHES:

1. Stand with left side toward wall at arm's length. Place palm flat against the wall at shoulder height.

2. Bend your knees slightly bringing your right foot in front of you, heel on the floor, foot flexed and toes pointing toward ceiling.

3. Lean slightly forward, looking straight ahead.

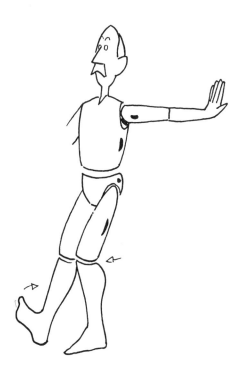

4. Hold this position for 4 seconds.

5. Return to starting position.

6. Keeping your knees together, bend your right leg backward, flex your foot and try to touch your bottom with your heel.

7. Hold this position for 4 seconds.

8. Do this sequence 4 times.

9. Turn around and repeat this exercise on the other side.

LEVEL II
CALF STRETCHES:

1. Stand with left side toward wall at arm's length. Place palm flat against the wall at shoulder height.

2. Bend your knees slightly bringing your right foot in front of you, heel on the floor, foot flexed and toes pointing toward ceiling.

3. Lean slightly forward, looking straight ahead.

4. Hold this position for 4 seconds.

5. Return to starting position.

6. Keeping your knees together, bend your right leg backward, flex your foot and try to touch your bottom with your heel.

7. Hold this position for 4 seconds.

8. Do this sequence 5 times.

9. Turn around and repeat this exercise on the other side.

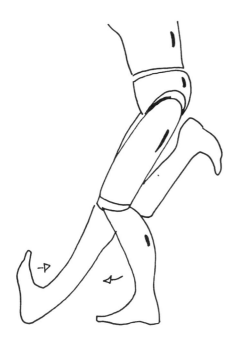

LEVEL III
CALF STRETCHES:

1. Stand with left side toward wall at arm's length. Place palm flat against the wall at shoulder height.

2. Bend your knees slightly bringing your right foot in front of you, heel on the floor, foot flexed and toes pointing toward ceiling.

3. Lean slightly forward, looking straight ahead.

4. Hold this position for 5 seconds.

5. Return to starting position.

6. Keeping your knees together, bend your right leg backward, flex your foot and try to touch your bottom with your heel.

7. Hold this position for 5 seconds.

8. Do this sequence 5 times.

9. Turn around and repeat this exercise on the other side.

Remember:
- do this exercise slowly

COOL-DOWN: LET'S STRETCH!

SESSION 4 - LEVEL I
SPINAL TWISTS II:

1. Lie on your back, bend knees toward chest, feet off the floor, and arms out to the sides.

2. Slowly roll knees to right side releasing left shoulder from floor.

3. Stretch and hold this position for 4 seconds.

4. Return to starting position.

5. Repeat this exercise to left side.

6. Do this sequence 4 times.

LEVEL II
SPINAL TWISTS II:

1. Lie on your back, bend knees toward chest, feet off the floor, and arms out to the sides.

2. Slowly roll knees to right side releasing left shoulder from floor.

3. Hold this position for 4 seconds.

4. Return to starting position.

5. Repeat this exercise to left side.

6. Do this sequence 5 times.

Level I + II

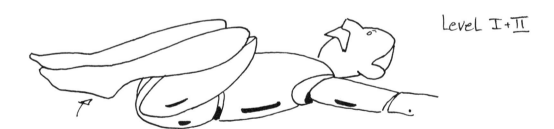

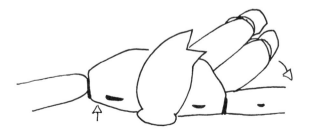

LEVEL III
SPINAL TWISTS II:

1. Lie on your back, both knees bent, feet flat on the floor.

2. Slowly roll knees to right side *keeping your left shoulder on the floor.*

3. Hold this position for 5 seconds.

4. Return to starting position.

5. Repeat this exercise to left side.

6. Do this sequence 5 times.

Remember:

- do not force these positions
- do this exercise slowly and smoothly

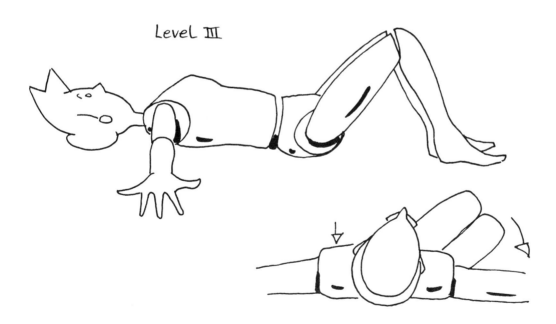

Level III

COOL-DOWN: LET'S RELAX!

SESSION 4 - LEVEL I

READ THE COMPLETE
RELAXATION EXERCISE
BEFORE YOU BEGIN

TOTAL TIME: 4 minutes

1. Turn on soft background music.

2. Lie on your back and cover yourself with a warm blanket.

3. Place your hands on your stomach.

4. Slowly breathe in through your nose so that your hands go up.

5. Slowly breathe out through your mouth, pulling your stomach in (your hands should go down).

6. Continue this slow breathing until you feel completely relaxed.

7. Let this relaxed feeling flow through your body — ENJOY.

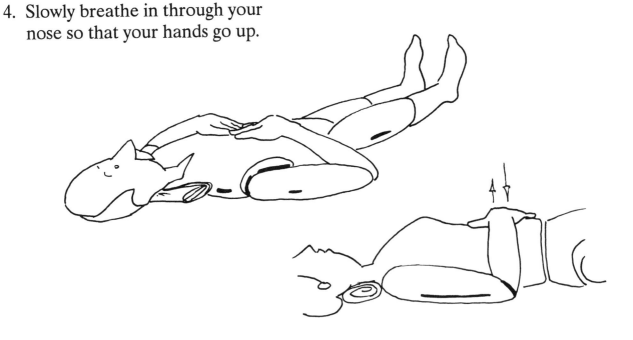

LEVEL II
Do Level I

LEVEL III
Do Level I

Remember:

- if possible, turn off some of the lights where you will be relaxing

- relax in a quiet area

- keep your breathing slow and rhythmic

- close your eyes when relaxing

- if you have a sleeping bag, use it rather than a blanket — it is excellent for these exercises

- be aware of the difference in your muscles when they are tensed or relaxed

- use a towel or a small pillow at the nape of your neck for support

- if you have lower back problems support your legs on the seat of a chair

LET'S GET FIT - SESSION 5

WARM-UP: LET'S BEGIN!

SESSION 5 - LEVEL I

TOTAL TIME: 4 minutes

PUT ON SOME LIVELY MUSIC.

1. Walk on the spot bringing knees toward chest at a slow, relaxed pace for 30 seconds.

2. Continue bringing knees toward chest and do the following movements for 30 seconds each:

a) slap knees

b) hands on shoulders, elbow circles

c) move your arms as if to swim (breast stroke)

d) lift knees to the side

e) swing right arm above head, then left

f) lift one leg in front, one behind

g) gradually, step more slowly

3. Stretch both arms above your head and breathe in deeply (3 times).

LEVEL II	LEVEL III
Do Level I.	Do Level I.

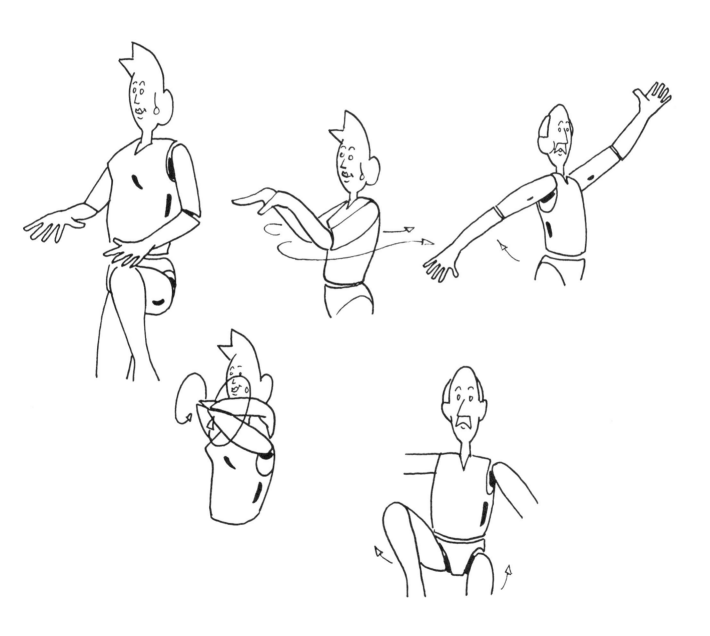

WARM-UP: LET'S LOOSEN UP!

SESSION 5 - LEVEL I ALPHABETS:

1. Write the first letter of your name with your head moving from left to right.

2. Write this letter 4 times.

3. Repeat moving from right to left.

LEVEL II ALPHABETS:

1. Place your arms down along the sides of your body, press heels of hands toward the floor. Keep this tension in your arms and...

2. Write your first name with your head moving from left to right.

3. Do this 4 times.

4. Do this sequence moving from right to left.

LEVEL III ALPHABETS:

1. Place your arms down along the sides of your body, press heels of hands toward the floor. Keep this tension in your arms and...

2. Write your first name with your head moving from left to right.

3. Do this 6 times.

4. Do this sequence moving from right to left.

Remember:

- do not arch back
- make large letters!

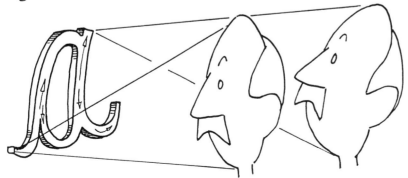
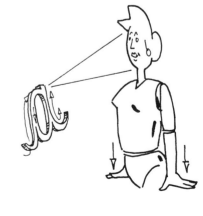

WARM-UP: LET'S LOOSEN UP!

SESSION 5 - LEVEL I
VOWELS ALOUD:

1. Slowly pronounce each of the vowels (A, E, I, O, U), exaggerating them as you say them out loud.

2. Do this sequence 4 times.

LEVEL II
VOWELS ALOUD:

1. Pull your chin inward.

2. Slowly pronounce each of the vowels (A, E, I, O, U), exaggerating them as you say them out loud.

3. Do this sequence 4 times.

LEVEL III
VOWELS ALOUD:

1. Pull your chin inward.

2. Slowly pronounce each of the vowels (A, E, I, O, U), exaggerating them as you say them out loud.

3. Do this sequence 6 times.

Remember:

- open your mouth wide for each vowel

- no one can see you, so stretch your face!

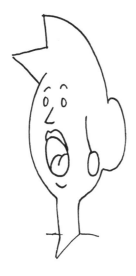

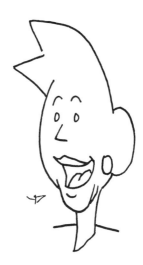

WARM-UP: LET'S LOOSEN UP!

SESSION 5 - LEVEL I
CROSSOVERS:

1. Slowly cross arms in front of your body at waist level.

2. Slowly uncross arms swinging them to the sides of your body.

3. Do this sequence 4 times.

4. Repeat this sequence with arms crossing behind you.

LEVEL II
CROSSOVERS:

1. Slowly cross arms in front of body at hip level.

2. Uncross arms and bring them straight out to the sides.

3. Repeat exercise, slowly bringing arms to cross at waist level, shoulder level, and above head.

4. Repeat this exercise in the opposite direction.

5. Do this sequence 4 times.

6. Move arms behind back so that arms cross.

7. Slowly cross and uncross arms behind body 4 times.

8. Relax.

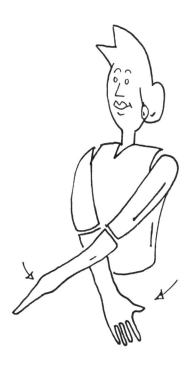

LEVEL III
CROSSOVERS:

1. Slowly cross arms in front of body at hip level.

2. Uncross arms and bring them straight out to the sides.

3. Repeat exercise, slowly bringing arms to cross at waist level, shoulder level and above head.

4. Repeat this exercise in the opposite direction.

5. Do this sequence 6 times.

6. Move arms behind back so that arms cross.

7. Slowly cross and uncross arms behind body 6 times.

8. Relax.

Remember:

- do not arch back

- do this slowly and smoothly — do not jerk!

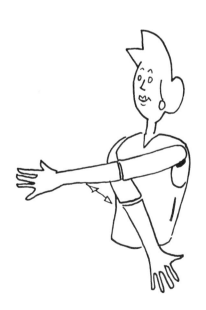
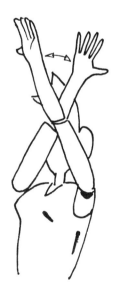
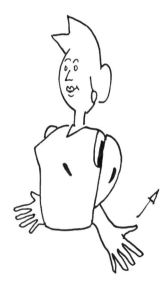

WARM-UP: LET'S LOOSEN UP!

SESSION 5 - LEVEL I
WRIST CIRCLES:

1. With palms facing ceiling, make a fist with both hands.

2. Describe circles with both fists keeping forearms still.

3. Complete 4 circles.

4. Repeat in opposite direction.

LEVEL II
WRIST CIRCLES:

1. Extend fingers of both hands.

2. Describe a circle with both hands, keeping forearms still.

3. Complete 4 circles.

4. Repeat in opposite direction.

LEVEL III
WRIST CIRCLES:

1. Extend fingers of both hands.

2. Describe a circle with both hands, keeping forearms still.

3. Complete 6 circles.

4. Repeat in opposite direction.

Remember:

- try to keep forearms still — the action is in the wrist!

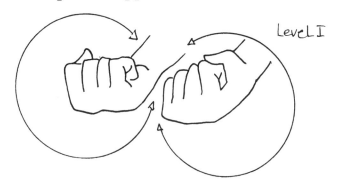

Level I

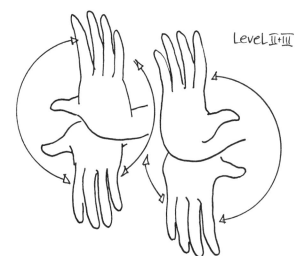

Level II + III

WARM-UP: LET'S LOOSEN UP!

SESSION 5 - LEVEL I
FINGER CURLS:

1. Spread the fingers of both hands as far apart as possible.

2. Turn palms to face ceiling.

3. Touch fingertips to upper palm.

4. Touch fingertips to middle palm.

5. Touch fingertips to lower palm.

6. Spread fingers apart.

7. Do this sequence 4 times.

LEVEL II
FINGER CURLS:

1. Place a sheet of paper (a paper towel) in each hand, arms straight out in front of body at shoulder level.

2. Crumple the paper, trying to form a small ball.

3. Do this sequence 4 times.

LEVEL III
FINGER CURLS:

1. Place a sheet of paper (a paper towel) in each hand, arms straight out in front of body at shoulder level.

2. Crumple the paper, trying to form a small ball.

3. Do this sequence 6 times.

Remember:

- use only your fingers to crumple the paper

Level II + III

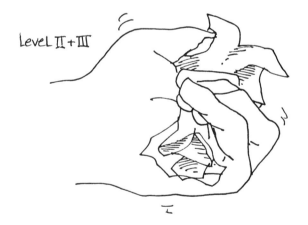

Level I

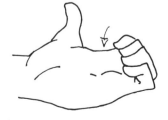

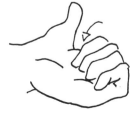

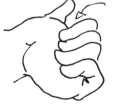

WARM-UP: LET'S LOOSEN UP!

SESSION 5 - LEVEL I
WAIST STRETCHES:

1. Place left arm behind you on lower back.

2. Raise right arm above head.

3. Turn to your left to look behind you.

4. Return to starting position.

5. Repeat on the other side.

6. Do this sequence 4 times.

Level I

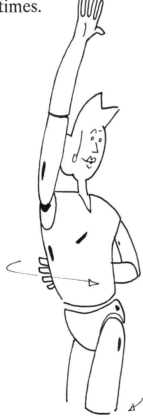

LEVEL II
WAIST STRETCHES:

1. Stand approximately 1 foot away from the wall, back toward the wall.

2. Place left arm behind you on lower back.

3. Raise right arm above head.

4. Twisting your upper body to the left, turn to look behind you, trying to place your right hand on the wall.

5. Return to starting position.

6. Repeat this exercise on the other side.

7. Do this sequence 4 times.

LEVEL III
WAIST STRETCHES:

1. Stand approximately 1 foot away from the wall, back toward the wall.

2. Place left arm behind you on lower back.

3. Raise right arm above head.

4. Twisting your upper body to the left, turn to look behind you, trying to place your right hand on the wall.

6. Return to starting position.

7. Repeat this exercise on the other side.

8. Do this sequence 6 times.

Remember:

- do not arch back

- do not lock knees

- keep this movement slow and smooth

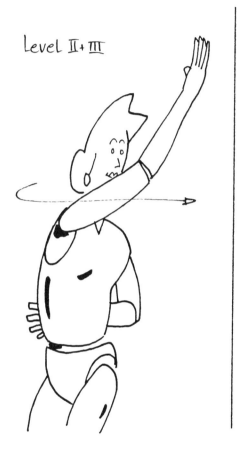

Level II + III

WARM UP: LET'S LOOSEN UP!

SESSION 5 - LEVEL I
LEG CIRCLES:

1. Stand with left side toward the wall at arm's length. Place palm of hand flat against the wall at shoulder height.

2. Slowly lift right leg to knee height in the front and describe a semicircle with 'lifting' leg going to the side and then to the back.

3. Repeat describing a semi-circle from back to front.

4. Return to starting position.

5. Do this sequence 4 times.

6. Turn around, place opposite hand on wall.

7. Repeat exercise with left leg.

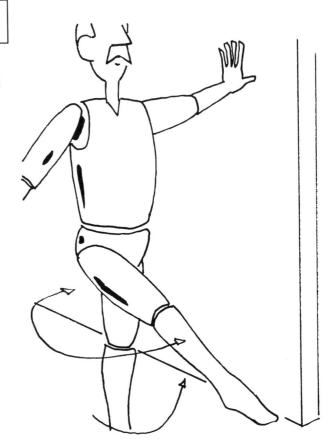

LEVEL II
LEG CIRCLES:

1. Stand with left side toward the wall at arm's length. Place palm flat against the wall at shoulder height.

2. Slowly lift right leg to knee height, crossing in front of left leg.

3. Describe a semicircle with 'lifting' leg going to the side and crossing behind left leg.

4. Repeat this movement from back to front.

5. Return to starting position.

6. Do this sequence 4 times.

7. Turn around, place opposite hand on wall.

8. Repeat exercise with left leg.

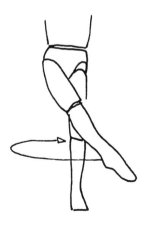

LEVEL III
LEG CIRCLES:

1. Stand with left side toward the wall at arm's length. Place palm flat against the wall at shoulder height.

2. Slowly lift right leg to knee height, crossing in front of left leg.

3. Describe a semicircle with 'lifting' leg going to the side and crossing behind left leg.

4. Repeat this movement from back to front.

5. Return to starting position.

6. Do this sequence 6 times.

7. Turn around, place opposite hand on wall.

8. Repeat exercise with left leg.

Remember:
- do not arch back — especially when bringing leg behind you
- stand up straight

WARM UP: LET'S LOOSEN UP!

SESSION 5 - LEVEL I
ANKLE CIRCLES:

1. Stand with left side toward the wall at arm's length. Place palm flat against the wall at shoulder height.

2. Bend right knee and lift right foot just off the floor.

3. Point your toes and describe 4 circles with your foot.

4. Repeat exercise, reversing the direction of the circles.

5. Turn around, place opposite hand on wall.

6. Repeat exercise with left foot.

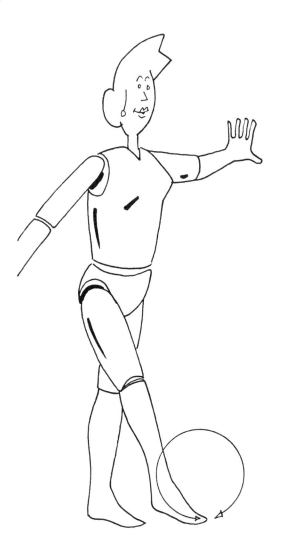

LEVEL II
ANKLE CIRCLES:

1. Stand with left side toward the wall at arm's length. Place palm flat against the wall at shoulder height.

2. Bend right knee and lift right foot just off the floor.

3. Point your toes and *very slowly* describe 6 *large* circles with your foot.

4. Repeat exercise, reversing the direction of the circles.

5. Turn around, place opposite hand on wall.

6. Repeat exercise with left foot.

LEVEL III
ANKLE CIRCLES:

1. Stand with left side toward the wall at arm's length. Place palm flat against the wall at shoulder height.

2. Bend right knee and lift right foot just off the floor.

3. Point your toes and *very slowly* describe 8 *large* circles with your foot.

4. Repeat exercise, reversing the direction of the circles.

5. Turn around, place opposite hand on wall.

6. Repeat exercise with left foot.

BODY OF THE CLASS: LET'S ENERGIZE!

SESSION 5 - LEVEL I

TOTAL TIME: 7 minutes

PUT ON SOME UPBEAT MUSIC.

WHILE STANDING, DO THE FOLLOWING MOVEMENTS FOR 30 SECONDS EACH:

1. Walk on the spot.

2. March, lifting knees and swinging arms.
   ✱

3. Continue marching, swim with your arms (the crawl).
   ✱

4. Lift right leg to the side, then left leg, swinging arms side to side.

5. Walk on the spot.

6. Lift legs side to side while touching elbow to knee.

7. March, swinging arms .

BODY CHECK - SING!

8. Repeat steps 3 — 7.
   ✱

9. Walk on the spot.

10. Step side to side.

Stretch both arms above your head and breathe in deeply (4 times).

BODY CHECK - MONITOR HEART RATE!

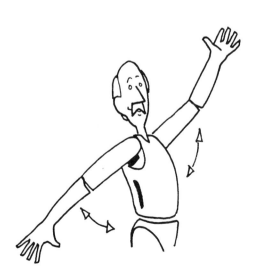

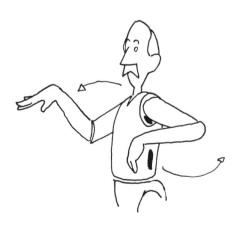

LEVEL II

TOTAL TIME: 8 minutes

Do Level I and when you come to an * add a march with a hop for 30 seconds.

LEVEL III

TOTAL TIME: 10 minutes

Do Level I and when you come to an * add a march with a hop, swinging your arms for 1 minute.

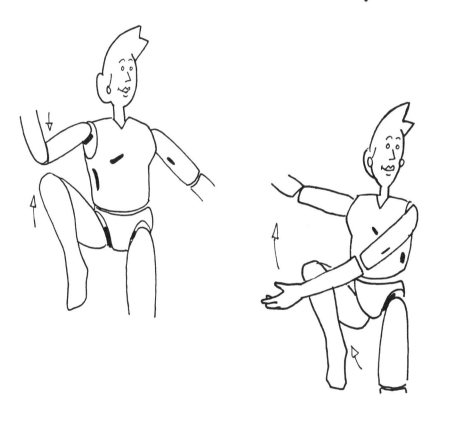
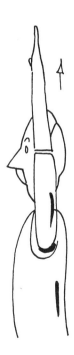

BODY OF THE CLASS: LET'S TONE UP!

SESSION 5 - LEVEL I
ARM CIRCLES: Sets: 3

Imagine that a large elastic band is around your wrists and is pulling your arms toward the ceiling — pull against this force!

1. Place your arms along the sides of your body, wrists flexed, palms facing floor.

2. Keeping arms stretched, describe 8 small circles with your arms starting close to the body and slowly raising your arms sideways until they are raised above your head (remember the elastic band!).

3. Reverse, bringing arms down alongside your body (remember the elastic band!).

4. Rest.

5. Complete the required number of sets.

LEVEL II
ARM CIRCLES: Sets: 3

With your weights around your wrists, do Level I .

LEVEL III
ARM CIRCLES: Sets: 3

With your weights around your wrists, do Level I .

Remember:

- do not arch back
- keep this movement slow and smooth
- do not forget to breathe
- keep knees slightly bent when doing this exercise

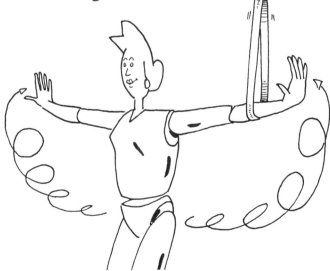

BODY OF THE CLASS: LET'S TONE UP!

SESSION 5 - LEVEL I
UP AND OVERS: Sets: 3

1. With your arms straight out in front of you at shoulder level, palms up, make tight fists and...

2. While breathing out, bring fists to touch shoulders (as if to lift a heavy object) (count 1,2,3).

3. While breathing in, slowly return to starting position (count 1,2,3).

4. Stretch arms above your head, elbows straight, palms facing forward.

5. Slowly bend arms so that hands touch your upper back (count 1,2,3).

6. Slowly stretch arms above your head (count 1,2,3).

7. Return to starting position (count 1,2,3).

8. Do this sequence 8 times.

9. Rest.

10. Complete the required number of sets.

LEVEL II
UP AND OVERS: Sets: 3

With your weights around your wrists, do Level I .

LEVEL III
UP AND OVERS: Sets: 3

With your weights around your wrists, do Level I .

Remember:

- do not arch back
- keep this movement slow and smooth
- keep knees slightly bent when doing this exercise

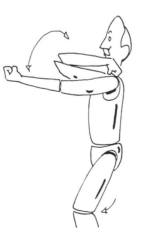
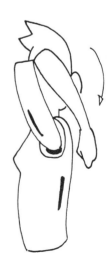

BODY OF THE CLASS: LET'S TONE UP!

SESSION 5 - LEVEL I
TUMMY TIGHTENERS: Sets: 3

1. Lie on your back, bend knees with your feet flat on the floor.

2. Place hands on thighs.

3. While breathing out, slowly raise head and both shoulder blades slightly off the floor (count 1,2,3).

4. While breathing in, slowly lower shoulders to the floor (count 1,2,3).

5. Do this sequence 4 times.

6. Rest.

7. Complete the required numbers of sets.

LEVEL II
TUMMY TIGHTENERS: Sets: 3

1. Lie on your back, bend knees with your feet flat on the floor.

2. Place hands on thighs.

3. While breathing out, slowly raise head and upper body off the floor making sure that *only* your waist remains on the floor (count 1,2,3).

4. While breathing in, slowly lower shoulders to the floor (count 1,2,3).

5. Do this sequence 4 times.

6. Rest.

7. Complete the required numbers of sets.

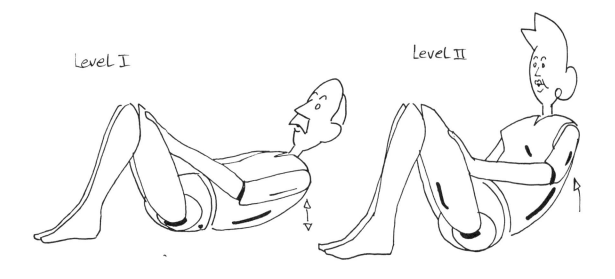

Level I   Level II

LEVEL III
TUMMY TIGHTENERS: Sets: 3

1. Lie on your back, bend knees with feet flat on the floor.

2. Place fingers on temples.

3. While breathing out, slowly raise head and upper body off the floor making sure that *only* your waist remains on the floor (count 1,2,3).

4. While breathing in, slowly lower shoulders to the floor (count 1,2,3).

5. Do this sequence 4 times.

6. Rest.

7. Complete the required numbers of sets.

Remember:

- make sure that shoulders touch the floor after each curl up

- raise both shoulder blades

- if you have difficulty keeping your feet on the floor, place weights around your ankles

- do not attempt to do a full sit up

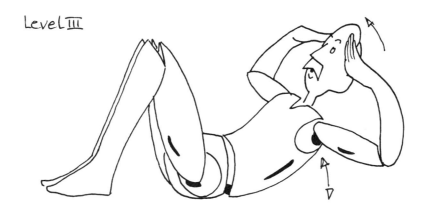

Level III

BODY OF THE CLASS: LET'S TONE UP!

SESSION 5 - LEVEL I
SWAYIN' SQUEEZES: Sets 3

1. Lie on your back, bend knees with your feet flat on the floor and shoulder width apart.

2. Lift your hips so that your bottom is slightly off the floor.

3. While squeezing your bottom, slowly sway your hips to the right and then to the left.

4. Slowly lower your bottom to the floor.

5. Do this sequence 4 times.

6. Rest.

7. Complete the required number of sets.

LEVEL II
SWAYIN' SQUEEZES: Sets 3

1. Lie on your back, bend knees with your feet flat on the floor, knees and feet together.

2. Lift your hips so that your bottom is slightly off the floor.

3. Squeeze your bottom and inner thighs tightly (count 1,2,3).

4. Keeping this squeeze, slowly sway hips to the right and then to the left.

5. Slowly lower your bottom to the floor (count 1,2,3).

6. Do this sequence 4 times.

7. Rest.

8. Complete the required number of sets.

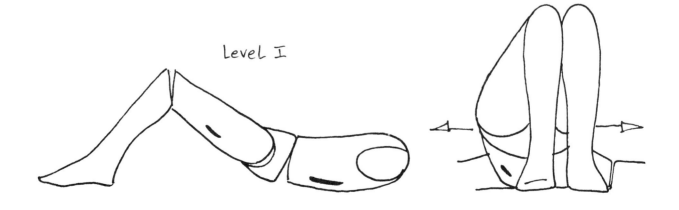

Level I

LEVEL III
SWAYIN' SQUEEZES: Sets 3

1. Lie on your back, bend knees with feet flat on the floor, knees and feet together.

2. Lift your hips so that your bottom is slightly off the floor.

3. Squeeze your bottom and inner thighs tightly (count 1,2,3).

4. Keeping this squeeze, slowly sway hips to the right and then to the left.

5. Slowly lower your bottom *almost* to the floor (count 1,2,3).

6. Raise hips once again.

7. Do this sequence 4 times.

8. Rest.

9. Complete the required number of sets.

Remember:
- do not arch back
- keep this movement slow and smooth
- do not forget to breathe

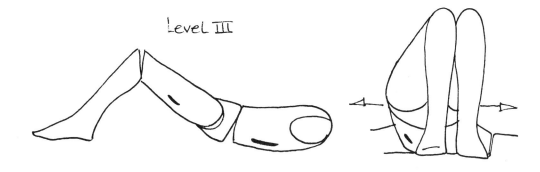

Level III

BODY OF THE CLASS: LET'S TONE UP!

SESSION 5 - LEVEL I
SIDE-TO-SIDE SWINGS: Sets: 3

1. Sit on the floor, back straight, right leg outstretched and left knee bent.

2. Place hands on floor behind you.

3. Flex your right foot so that toes are pointing toward the ceiling (tighten your thigh muscles).

4. Keeping muscles tightened, slowly lift right leg until heel is approximately 1 foot off the floor.

5. *Slowly* swing it to your right side.

6. Without touching the floor, bring your leg back to the centre.

7. Slowly lower leg to the floor.

8. Repeat this exercise with your left leg.

9. Do this sequence 4 times.

10. Rest.

11. Complete the required number of sets.

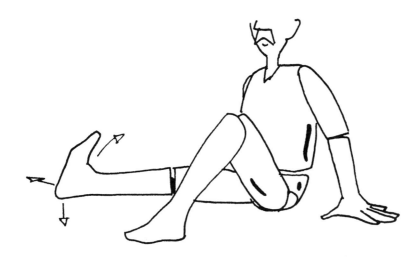

LEVEL II
SIDE-TO-SIDE SWINGS: Sets: 3

With your weights around your ankles, do Level I.

LEVEL III
SIDE-TO-SIDE SWINGS: Sets: 3

With your weights around your ankles, do Level I.

Remember:

- keep this movement slow and smooth
- do not forget to breathe

BODY OF THE CLASS: LET'S TONE UP!

SESSION 5 - LEVEL I
THE PENDULUM: Sets: 3

1. Lie on your left side, head resting on left arm, legs in straight line with your upper body.

2. With toes pointed, lift your right leg as high as possible, keeping hips facing forward.

3. Slowly bring your right foot in front of you to touch the floor.

4. Raise your right leg in front.

5. Raise and lower right leg in front of you 4 times.

6. Raise right leg once again, return it to the side and lower it to rest on left leg.

7. Rest.

8. Complete the required number of sets.

9. Turn over so that you lie on your right side.

10. Repeat this exercise with your left leg.

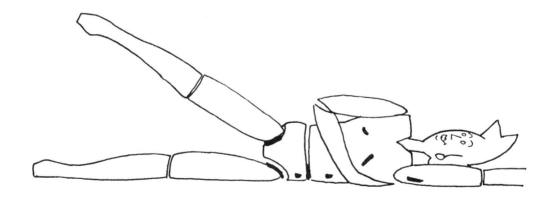

LEVEL II
THE PENDULUM: Sets: 3

With your weights around your ankles, do Level I.

LEVEL III
THE PENDULUM: Sets: 3

With your weights around your ankles, do Level I.

Remember:

- do not arch back
- keep upper body still when lifting leg
- use hand on floor in front of you for support
- keep this movement slow and smooth
- do not forget to breathe

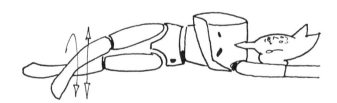

COOL-DOWN: LET'S STRETCH!

SESSION 5 - LEVEL I
ARM STRETCHES:

1. Lift your arms toward the ceiling.

2. Grab your right elbow with your left hand.

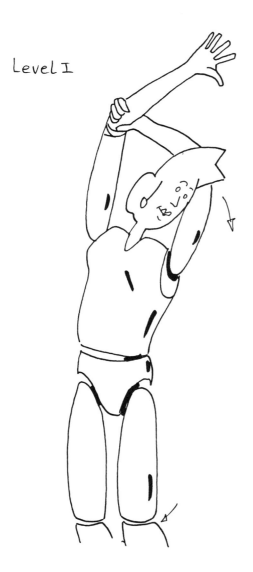

Level I

3. Lean body to the left with your left hand pulling on right elbow (feel the stretch on your right side).

4. Stretch and hold this position for 4 seconds.

5. Return to **BASIC POSITION**.

6. Repeat this exercise to right side.

7. Do this sequence 5 times.

LEVEL II
ARM STRETCHES:

1. Lift your arms toward the ceiling, fold them and rest them on top of your head.

2. With left hand pulling on right elbow, lean body to the left. Let left elbow become heavy, pulling your upper body down.

3. Stretch and hold this position for 4 seconds.

4. Return to starting position.

5. Repeat this exercise to left side.

6. Do this sequence 6 times.

LEVEL III
ARM STRETCHES:

1. Lift your arms toward the ceiling.

2. Grab your right wrist with your left hand.

3. Lean body to the left with your left hand pulling on your right wrist (feel the stretch on your right side).

4. Stretch and hold this position for 5 seconds.

5. Return to **BASIC POSITION**.

6. Repeat this exercise to right side.

7. Do this sequence 6 times.

Remember:

- do not arch back

- keep knees slightly bent when doing this exercise

- do this exercise slowly

- always bend directly to the side, not forward or backward

- keep hips facing forward

- this exercise can be done while sitting on a chair or with your back against the wall

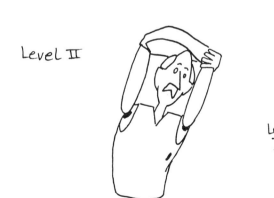

Level II

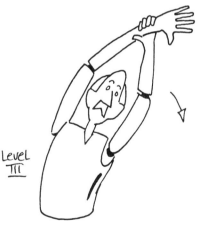

Level III

COOL-DOWN: LET'S STRETCH!

SESSION 5 - LEVEL I
PYRAMID STRETCH:

1. Place hands on shoulders and bring elbows in front of body to touch.

2. Stretch and hold this position for 4 seconds.

3. Swing left elbow up toward the ceiling and right elbow down toward the floor.

4. Gently pull elbows toward the back.

5. Stretch and hold this position for 4 seconds.

6. Repeat this exercise, switching elbows.

7. Do this sequence 5 times.

LEVEL II
PYRAMID STRETCH:

1. Stretch your arms out in front of you, palms facing each other.

2. Keeping arms stretched, slowly swing your right arm up and back over your head while your left arm slowly swings down and back.

3. Stretch and hold this position for 4 seconds.

4. Cross arms in front of body, keeping arms straight.

5. Stretch and hold this position for 4 seconds.

6. Repeat this exercise, swinging left arm up and right arm down to start.

7. Do this sequence 6 times.

Level I

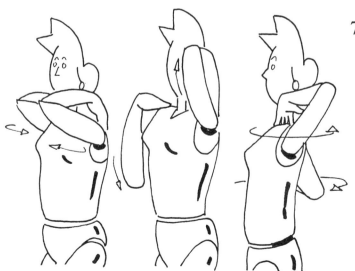

LEVEL III
PYRAMID STRETCH:

1. Stretch your arms out in front of you, palms facing each other.

2. Keeping arms stretched, slowly swing your right arm up and back over your head while your left arm slowly swings down and back.

3. Stretch and hold this position for 5 seconds.

4. Cross arms in front of body, keeping them straight.

5. Stretch and hold this position for 5 seconds.

6. Repeat this exercise, swinging left arm up and right arm down to start.

7. Do this sequence 6 times.

Remember:
- do not arch back
- keep knees slightly bent when doing this exercise
- do this exercise slowly

Level II

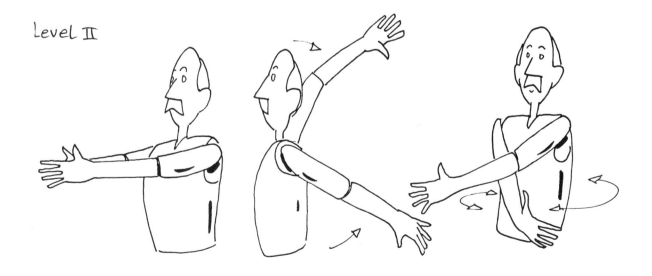

COOL-DOWN: LET'S STRETCH!

SESSION 5 - LEVEL I
KNEE DROPS:

1. Stand with left side toward the wall at arm's length. Place palm flat against the wall at shoulder height.

2. Take a big step forward with your right foot, keeping left leg straight, heel on the floor, right knee bent.

3. Bend left knee, trying to keep heel on the floor.

4. Hold this position for 4 seconds.

5. Keeping feet in this position, stand up straight (straighten knees).

6. Flex right foot so that toes are pointing toward the ceiling, bend left knee.

7. Hold this position for 4 seconds.

8. Return to **BASIC POSITION** .

9. Do this sequence 5 times.

10. Turn around and repeat this exercise on the other side.

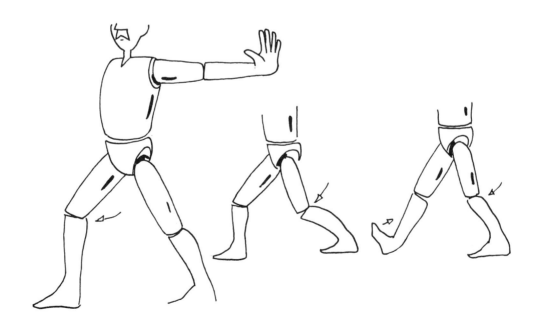

LEVEL II
KNEE DROPS:

1. Stand with left side toward the wall at arm's length. Place palm of hand flat against the wall at shoulder height.

2. Take a big step forward with your right foot, keeping left leg straight, heel on the floor, right knee bent.

3. Bend left knee, trying to keep heel on the floor.

4. Hold this position for 4 seconds.

5. Keeping feet in this position, stand up straight (straighten knees).

6. Flex right foot so that toes are pointing toward the ceiling, bend left knee.

7. Hold this position for 4 seconds.

8. Return to **BASIC POSITION**.

9. Do this sequence 6 times.

10. Turn around and repeat this exercise on the other side.

LEVEL III
KNEE DROPS:

1. Stand with left side toward the wall at arm's length. Place palm of hand flat against the wall at shoulder height.

2. Take a big step forward with your right foot, keeping left leg straight, heel on the floor, right knee bent.

3. Bend left knee, trying to keep heel on the floor.

4. Hold this position for 5 seconds.

5. Keeping feet in this position, stand up straight (straighten knees).

6. Flex right foot so that toes are pointing toward the ceiling, bend left knee.

7. Hold this position for 5 seconds.

8. Return to **BASIC POSITION**.

9. Do this sequence 6 times.

10. Turn around and repeat this exercise on the other side.

Remember:

- do this exercise slowly

COOL DOWN: LET'S STRETCH!

SESSION 5 - LEVEL I
LIFT AND REACH:

1. Lie on your back, knees bent, feet flat on the floor, arms out to the side.

2. Lift right leg straight up in the air.

3. Cross right leg over to left side and try to touch the floor. Release your right shoulder from the floor.

4. Reach and hold this position for 4 seconds.

5. Return to starting position.

6. Repeat this exercise with left leg.

7. Do this sequence 5 times.

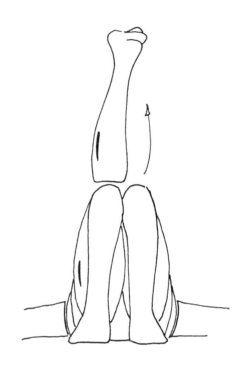

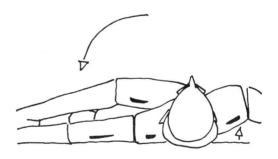

LEVEL II
LIFT AND REACH:

1. Lie on your back, knees bent, feet flat on the floor, arms out to the side.

2. Lift right leg straight up in the air.

3. Cross right leg over to left side and try to touch the floor. Release your right shoulder from the floor.

4. Slide right foot along floor to meet left hand.

5. Hold this position for 4 seconds.

6. Return to starting position.

7. Repeat this exercise with left leg.

8. Do this sequence 6 times.

LEVEL III
LIFT AND REACH:

1. Lie on your back, knees bent, feet flat on the floor, arms out to the side.

2. Lift right leg straight up in the air.

3. Cross right leg over to left side and try to touch the floor, *keeping your right shoulder on the floor.*

4. Bring your right foot up to your left hand and grab your toes.

5. Hold this position for 5 seconds.

6. Return to starting position.

7. Repeat this exercise with your left leg.

8. Do this sequence 6 times.

Remember:

- do not force these positions

- do this exercise slowly and smoothly

Level II

Level III

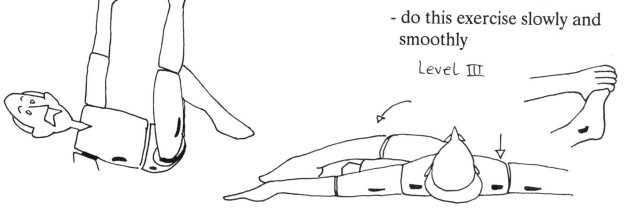

COOL DOWN: LET'S RELAX!

SESSION 5 - LEVEL I

TOTAL TIME: 4 minutes

READ THE <u>COMPLETE</u>
RELAXATION EXERCISE
BEFORE YOU BEGIN

This relaxation should take approximately 4 minutes to complete.

1. Turn on soft background music.

2. Lie on your back and cover yourself with a warm blanket.

3. Tighten your calf muscles, hold for 3 seconds and relax.

4. Repeat this contraction and relaxation for the following parts of your body:

   thighs, stomach, bottom, shoulders, arms, hands, face.

5. Breathe slowly until your body is completely relaxed.

6. Continue this slow breathing until you feel completely relaxed.

7. Let this relaxed feeling flow through your body — ENJOY.

LEVEL II

Do Level I .

LEVEL III

Do Level I .

Remember:

- if possible, turn off some of the lights where you will be relaxing

- relax in a quiet area

- keep your breathing slow and rhythmic

- close your eyes when relaxing

- if you have a sleeping bag, use it rather than a blanket — it is excellent for these exercises

- be aware of the difference in your muscles when they are tensed and/or relaxed

- use a towel or a small pillow at the nape of your neck for support

- if you have lower back problems, support your legs on the seat of a chair

CHAPTER 7

HEALTHY, HAPPY AGING

Now that you have learned how good regular exercise can make you feel, you should begin to think of including fitness in your day-to-day living. In other words, THINK FIT! Being fit does not necessarily mean that you are able to run a marathon or even do all the things that you were able to do when you were young. Being fit simply means that you have the energy to carry on your day-to-day living with enjoyment and have enough pep left over to meet other energy demands. It is these other demands that bring enjoyment to our lives. These are the activities that bring us pleasure — gardening, golfing, walking, shopping, travelling or playing with your grandchildren. You can have this extra zest for life if exercise becomes a part of your routine. A regular exercise programme such as presented in this book is an excellent beginning; its benefits are obvious; just review Chapter 1 to understand what a positive impact physical activity has on the aging process. However, you should make a conscious effort to include physical activity in everything that you do. This will bring vigour and vitality to your life.

To add more activity to your day, all you have to do is try to avoid doing things the easy, effortless way. If you live on the second floor, don't take the elevator, walk up! If your favourite store is on the third floor, walk up; then double the pleasure — walk down!

Walking, many experts say, is the safest, most complete form of exercise. Walking requires no instruction; it can be done almost anywhere, at any time; it costs nothing, and most importantly, you can do it with a friend. Walk around your neighbourhood. Who knows who you will meet or what you may learn! Often the most pleasurable walks are those taken in the country or in a nearby park. Watch for birds, enjoy the fresh air, ease your frustrations and you will understand why many people say that a hike in the woods is better than any medication.

Take along a walking stick; it is excellent for poking the ground, checking the terrain and may even be useful if you become tired. A walking stick is not a sign of old age, merely a handy tool that dedicated hikers never leave behind.

Swimming is also an excellent form of exercise. Water has the capability of lessening the weight on your joints. What could be better than moving your body without the added problem of supporting your weight? Make sure that the water is warm — cold water causes your muscles to contract, thereby causing them to be less

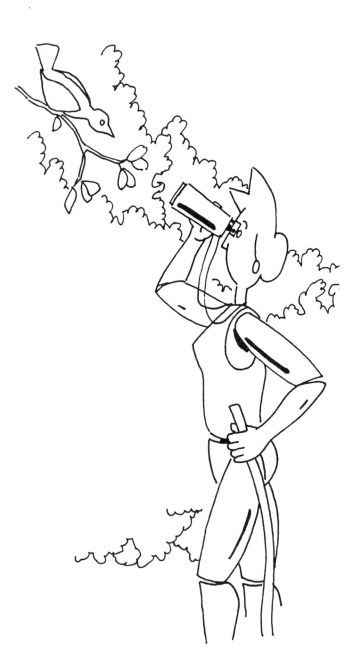

pliable. If you are not comfortable in deep water, stay in the shallow end and move your arms and legs through their full range of motion. Take along a friend and play with a beach ball. You'll be surprised at how effective and enjoyable this workout can be!

There are actually few sports that may be a risk for you. Remember, in the chapter "Exercising Safely" you were advised to try to eliminate fast, sharp, movements. Sports with these movements (e.g. basketball, racquet ball) could cause damage to the shoulder or knee. If you are used to playing these games, by all means continue — your body is conditioned to make these moves.

Don't forget dancing! You may not be Ginger Rogers or Fred Astaire, but the benefits of dancing far outweigh the embarrassment of missing a step or two. Dancing involves all the right things: an excellent workout for your heart, rhythm, balance, social interaction and enjoyable music. Join a club, even if you don't have a partner. Many groups today practise line dancing or dancing without partners. Join these groups — you'll be sure to meet several men or women who share similar interests and you're almost guaranteed to have fun!

There are many other ways to incorporate physical activity into your life. Some suggestions that might appeal to you:

1. While talking on the telephone:
   - move your fingers and toes to keep them limber

   - massage your feet by rolling a small bottle beneath them

   - practise your good breathing techniques (Chapter 6) while listening to the person on the other end

2. When shopping, walk around the mall once before you even enter a store.

3. In the winter when sidewalks are slippery, go to your local mall and do your walking there. You are sure to be kept busy watching the activity in the shopping centre.

4. Wash your own car in the summer. It's not only good exercise, it saves you money.

5. When you wake up in the morning, stretch every way that you can. Enjoy the feeling of waking up, it's a good way to start the day.

6. When sitting for long periods of time, be sure to take time for an 'exercise break'. Just by moving your body and your joints every 30 minutes, you can prevent the stiffness that often occurs from sitting still.

7. When knitting, crocheting or reading, every 30 minutes or so, put down what you're doing and move.

8. Go on a picnic with friends.

9. When travelling in a car, make frequent stops, get out of the car and enjoy the scenery by being a part of it.

10. Make relaxation exercises a part of your day. Practise them when you are upset, worried, or just need a change of pace.

11. Laugh several times a day. Laughter is an excellent exercise involving many body systems.

There are benefits to exercise other than just becoming physically fit. When you are active, the blood flow increases to all parts of the body, but most importantly to the brain. Physical activity can make you more alert. You will reduce your mental tiredness and sometimes the accompanying tension, strain and boredom. With this increased alertness there are many new tasks and interests on which you can focus.

What about:

- reading a new book

- learning a new hobby (you can do it, it just takes time)

- volunteering as a club executive

- learning more about your body

- becoming a story-teller at a local school or library

- getting a part-time job

- learning more about our environmental issues

- writing letters to friends with whom you haven't communicated in a long time

- visit someone who is ill and actually cheer them up

- put together a book of your family history with pictures, stories and memorabilia — it will be a prized treasure!

There are other components of your life that must be addressed to make you the best that you can possibly be. We have discussed activity in terms of what it means to your body and mind. Another important part of healthy living is making sure that your body is properly nourished. Do not neglect proper eating habits! Refer to the chapter "Living with Aging" to review problems associated with eating habits as we age. Do keep Canada's Food Guide handy and refer to it often.

One other important thing to remember: form a partnership with your physician! Time and time again in this book we have reminded you to consult your physician. He/she

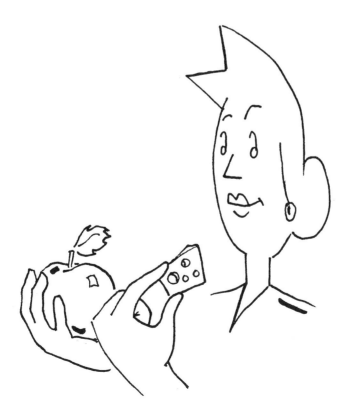

understands how your body works and the common disorders associated with aging. Keep your physician informed of the changes in your life so that you're on the same team. Isn't it more effective to have as many members on your team as possible? When you are physically fit in body and mind, when you eat well and when you have formed a strong partnership with your physician, you are well on your way to 'the good life'.

In this book we have explained how your body ages and how to bring life and vigour to your days. With physical activity you have the key to *healthy, happy aging*! The rest is up to you!

CHAPTER 8

FOR THE INSTRUCTOR

To be physically active is a natural human need. Every movement of the human body is a kind of physical activity. Some of these movements might be required for survival such as raising the arm to bring food up to the mouth to eat. Other movements are performed simply for the pleasure they bring; the person who decides to walk for the enjoyment of being outside is a good example.

A senior could be more inclined to become physically active if he/she believed that exercise provided either direct or indirect benefits.

For some people, exercising is a way of releasing daily stress; others might be interested in exercise to increase their level of well-being. In fact, there are as many reasons to exercise as there are people exercising.

Since reasons for exercising are numerous, a person may change his/her motives for doing so in a short period of time. A senior may start exercising so that he or she is in contact with other people and not alone at home. Later, that same senior may continue to exercise realizing that through a physical activity programme he/she is able to accomplish more things in the course of a day, leading to an improved quality of life.

There are seniors interested in exercising in every community. Being an instructor, your responsibility is to identify this group, to define its needs and to offer a programme that will be satisfactory and enjoyable to them. As an instructor, you have to bear in mind that organizing a general fitness programme might be an easy task but the challenge lies in ensuring this programme meets the needs and expectations of the seniors involved.

The following pages will introduce guidelines designed to help the instructor and programme planners accomplish the important task of planning and teaching a seniors' fitness programme, ensuring that it meets the needs and expectations of the participants.

Section 1

PLANNING A FITNESS PROGRAMME

The Pre-Programme Planning

This section will discuss different steps to follow in order to complete the set-up and planning of a fitness programme for seniors. We will discuss the administrative planning of the programme, elements such as determining the needs of the target group, consultation with fitness organizations such as community administration (e.g. the recreation department), with the institutions that might be involved, with specialists in the field of physical activity, the initial planning of the programme, the facilities, the material needed, the money involved, the personnel, publicity of the programme, the participants and the duration of the programme.

Determining The Needs Of The Target Group

The first step in planning a successful fitness programme is to consult the seniors themselves. When specific information has been gathered both on the facility and the future senior participants (expectations, capacity, etc.), it will be possible to design a more personalized fitness programme.

What Information Should Be Collected?

Content of the Programme:
What type of exercise is expected by the future participants? Simple exercises? Games, dances or pool exercises?

Frequency of the Programme:
When should the programme be offered? What day or days? What time? How long should the class last?

The answers to these questions will help you make some decisions. For example, you might decide that the programme should last eight weeks, be held three times per week — Monday, Wednesday and Friday starting at 10:30 am until 11:45 am.

Characteristics of the Participating Seniors

What is the average age of the seniors? What is the ratio of men/women? What is the average level of fitness of these seniors? What do the seniors like/dislike about physical activity? What are their motives for participating? What are their common interests?

Some of the things that you might learn from the answers to these questions: your class should be adapted to members of a certain senior citizens' club at a beginner level and should include cooperative games.

Facilities

Where should the programme be offered (if the community offers a choice)? Should the programme be offered indoors or outdoors? Should the programme be offered in a specialized room such as a gymnasium, swimming pool or all-purpose room? Before offering these choices to the future participants, the services available within the facilities should be investigated (showers, waiting room, washrooms, parking and so on). All these answers will help create an interesting atmosphere for the future senior participants.

Qualities of the Instructor

Should these leaders be the same age, younger or older than the participants? Which type of training should these leaders have: university training, college training, specialized fitness training, etc? What should the ratio of leader to participant be? Thus, the group might wish to use one of their peers as a leader and expect him/her to get some basic training in fitness. The group might, on the other hand, expect to be instructed by a university trained leader.

Expectations of the Participants

What do the seniors expect? Do they want to:

- improve their level of activity

- learn new techniques

- lose weight

- have fun

- socialize and participate in activities with their peers?

This groundwork is the base for the success of your fitness class and should be completed before developing your programme. This work lays the foundation for future tasks that will provide the technical answers to ensure the success of your programme.

Consultation With Fitness Organizations

A fitness organization is an organization that has expertise in one area and has received the mandate to advise people on how to practise certain physical activities, such as tennis or lawn bowling, both safely and correctly.

This guidance is necessary when rules have to be followed by everybody, e.g. tennis. These organizations also give advice on the best way to learn a new activity. For example, the Red Cross is available for consultation concerning the safest and most accepted method of teaching swimming.

Finally, there are some organizations that give advice on how programmes should be run in one area or another, on what to do and what to avoid. An example of such an organization is the Secretariat for Fitness in the Third Age.

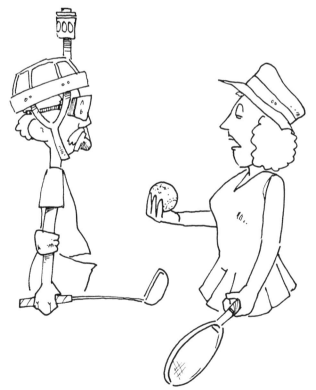

Consultation With Institutions

Institutions are organizations such as municipal recreation departments, private recreation organizations such as the YMCA, universities, colleges, hospitals (Élisabeth Bruyère Health Centre - Positive Health for Seniors), and private centres that specialize in offering physical activity programmes and have developed an expertise in this area.

By contacting them, you could benefit from their experience. You could discover that they are offering programmes with the exact characteristics you need for your programme. If not, these organizations might be interested in helping you develop a programme adapted to your group. Most of the time they will be happy to offer their assistance to help you plan your fitness programme.

Consultation With Specialists In The Field Of Physical Activity

A specialist is a person with a special training in the area of physical activity either as leader, planner or researcher. If possible, consult with at least one person in each category.

From these people, you may obtain information and material for your group on different aspects of physical activity. For example:

- teaching
- evaluation
- motivation
- rules of specific sports

This consultation process will make sure that your programme is up-to-date with the latest findings in the area of physical fitness and that you will offer the best programme available.

Planning Your Programme

The next step is planning the content of your programme. Once you have completed the consultation phases as outlined, you will be able to develop a series of objectives. Now you must decide upon:

- the content
- the leader
- when the classes will take place
- where the classes will be held
- the registration cost
- the budget

The following questions are designed to help you with planning your fitness programme.

What do you need for the programme and what did the seniors that you spoke to request? (showers, waiting room, washrooms, etc.)

Are there other programmes that could interfere with your fitness classes because of noise or other distractions?

Are there other leisure events that could interfere with the fitness programme (social events, trips, etc.)?

Is there a place where your materials and equipment could be stored?

Who will prepare material needed for the programme before it starts and who will put it back where it belongs? Involving participants in this activity could make this task easier.

Who will be responsible for cleaning the facility before and after the activities?

Are there enough parking spaces and/or is there good public transportation close by?

Is it possible to get medical help easily if necessary? Are the people in charge trained for emergencies?

Activity Room

Is it accessible (in a central location, stairs or elevators, wide doors for wheelchairs, etc.)?

Is it equipped with good lighting?

Is there a telephone and are there emergency telephone numbers available at all times?

Is the room clean, attractive and appropriate for the type of activities planned?

Is there a first aid kit available?

Is there a good ventilation system in the room? Is it adequate for the type of activities you are planning?

Is there room for the organizer(s) of the programme, visitors and spectators, to wait or watch without disturbing the group?

Are exercise mats available?

Equipment

What equipment will be provided by you or the facility, and what will the participants be expected to bring?

What steps must you follow to make sure that the equipment will be ready? What has to be bought? Delivered? Stored? Inventoried?

How can participants be told in advance that they will have to purchase equipment, e.g. shoes, towels, etc? What will the overall cost be for this equipment?

Do stores in the community have the equipment available that the participants are required to purchase, e.g. shoes, ball?

Are participants expected to rent equipment? How will this be handled?

What is the total cost for equipment? How much is paid by you, the facility or the participants?

Is the equipment safe?

Who will be responsible for repairing equipment after the programme has started?

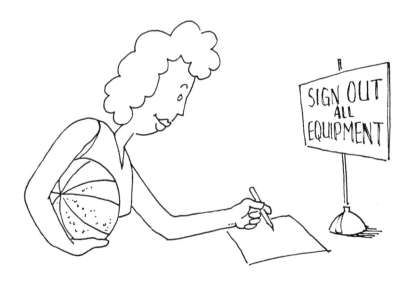

Budget

How will the programme be financed? How much money will be provided by you, by registration fees, sponsors, or a combination of the above?

What will you need to charge?

Is a registration fee to make sure that you do not go over budget?

Who will collect registration fees if there are any? Will receipts be issued?

How will participants pay their registration fees? Cash? Cheque? Credit card? Money order?

Will there be special fees, e.g. reduction for husband and wife, provision for seniors who are unable to afford the cost? Who will be eligible? How will you keep track of it?

Must the registration fee be paid in a lump sum or can interim payments be made? If so, how many payments? When will the last payment be? How will you keep track of this?

How will the registration fee for the programme be handled? Will it be deposited in the bank? Under whose name will the bank account be opened — your name or in the name of the sponsoring organization?

Who will approve expenses? Who will be responsible for the budget?

Will unsatisfied participants be eligible for a refund? If so, how will they be reimbursed and how much?

If a participant becomes ill and unable to continue, will they get a refund? If so, how much?

Personnel

Will you and other instructors be volunteers or paid a salary?

What qualities will you look for in another instructor? Qualifications? Experience? Attitude and aptitude? Language? Age?

Does this instructor have training in the area of the programme or will training need to be provided?

How will you decide who you will hire?

Publicity

What message do you want to convey to the public?

What kind of information would attract future participants?

Where will you reach future participants?

What is the best way to get the message across?

Will it be necessary to use more than one medium (newspaper, radio, television)? Why?

Who would be the best person to produce these advertisements?

What costs will be involved?

What is the time frame involved?

How can you field test this publicity to ensure it appeals to your target group?

Is there some way in which you can make your advertising more personal?

If your advertising is more successful than expected, will you be able to meet the demand?

Have you thought of having a day when each participant may bring a friend?

Participants

Will the group be heterogeneous (men and women) or homogeneous (men or women)?

Is it possible to prevent the formation of cliques inside the large group?

Will the programme allow for creativity and spontaneity from the group as well as from individuals?

Will the programme be designed so that activities can be varied to fulfill the different needs of your participants?

How will you make sure that future participants receive the correct information about the details of the programme?

Registration

Is the registration procedure uncomplicated and speedy?

Where will registration be held?

Will there be a cut-off date for registration?

Will there be registration criteria, e.g. maximum number of participants, participant's fitness level — beginner, intermediate, advanced?

Duration Of The Programme

How long will the programme last? How many times per week? How long will each class last? Twice a week for one hour?

Should there be time to socialize before or after exercising? How long? Perhaps every month a small lunch could be organized after class. The menu could be planned in such a way that it would help participants in their understanding of a healthy, nutritious diet while socializing with other members of the group.

Will the programme be interrupted by special events such as Christmas, Easter, summer and other holidays?

What effect will these interruptions have on the programme?

When is the best time of day to hold the class? Is there a time that the classes should not be held? For example, an exercise class should never be held immediately after a meal.

Are the types of activities planned influenced by the weather? How? What alternate plans can you make?

Will there be other groups using the facilities before or after your programme? What problems could arise?

How will cancellation of a class be handled, e.g. instructor illness, bad weather?

Section 2

PLANNING AND TEACHING A FITNESS CLASS

The next few pages will deal with points to consider when planning and presenting the exercises and activities involved in a fitness class. This section is divided into three sections: the pre-class preparation, the actual teaching of a class and the after class evaluation.

Preparation Before Class Begins

Before beginning your exercise class, it is important to think of what you want to achieve for the benefit of your participants. Goals and objectives will help you evaluate your programme.

What Is A Goal?

A goal is what you wish to achieve during your programme. You can decide on your goal after you have gathered information from your participants on the kind of activities they would like to have or need during class.

For example, the goal of a fitness programme could be to improve the level of aerobic fitness of the participants. This goal does not talk about the initial level of aerobic fitness of the participants or the level of aerobic fitness that is expected at the end of the programme. Nevertheless, it is precise enough to decide on the types of exercises that need to be introduced to improve the level of aerobic fitness of the participants.

What Are the Objectives?

An objective is an ideal to be reached and should be stated in such a way that it can be measured. For example, at the end of the programme every participant should be able to walk non-stop while talking with a partner for a distance of .6 miles (1 km) more than their present walking distance.

An objective can provide you with a plan of what is to be achieved at different stages of the programme, be it one class, one week, one month, or a full session of ten weeks.

Putting Your Class Together

PLANNING YOUR CLASS

The second step in planning a fitness programme is to choose the different activities for each class. The activities chosen must be related to the goals and objectives of the programme. Each class must have a similar activity pattern (see FIGURE 1).

Choosing The Right Order Of Exercises And Activities

Exercises and activities that are part of a fitness class should be introduced in a certain order. This gives you, the

FIGURE 1

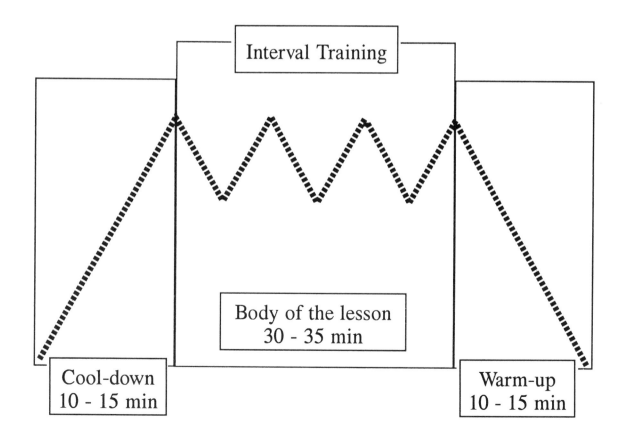

instructor, a simple way of making sure that you exercise every part of the body. During a fitness class, exercises for different parts of the body should be introduced in the following order:

1. Head, shoulders and neck.

2. Back and chest.

3. Arms, wrists and hands.

4. Abdomen, back and pelvis.

5. Legs and feet.

The Welcoming Period

The introduction or initial contact with the participants is extremely important. In some cases participants may have rushed to class or feel a bit anxious. A warm and quiet greeting will help participants make the transition to concentrate on exercise and the upcoming class.

It is also important to provide participants with information on the objectives or to present the material to be taught during the class.

Participants should be reminded about safety (working in pairs, wearing the proper exercise gear, etc.) and different warning signs (dizziness, shortness of breath, etc.).

**The Warm-Up
"LET'S BEGIN" and
"LET'S LOOSEN UP"**

The aim of the warm-up is to prepare your body physically and mentally to participate in the class activities.

The activities chosen for the warm-up are mostly non-violent and very progressive. A walk followed by some range of motion exercises, are good warm-up activities.

These activities will warm-up your large muscles and help prepare your body for exercise.

The warm-up period should last between 10 and 15 minutes.

An increase in your heart rate during the warm-up period is an indication that a larger amount of blood has begun to pump throughout your body. As a result, blood vessels in the lungs and muscles will begin to enlarge to accommodate this increase in blood flow. Now your body is ready to work harder and transport the extra blood pumped during vigorous exercise.

It is important for you to provide the participants with a chance to do some warm-up exercises by themselves.

In some cases, special exercises may have been prescribed to participants by their physicians to help a specific problem such as back pain, joint stiffness, or special exercises for the hips or knees.

A warm up will:

- gradually increase heart rate

- gradually increase breathing rate and by doing so, warm the muscles involved in breathing

- warm the muscles of the body making them more pliable

- increase the flow of blood to the muscles

- warm tendons, improving their ability to stretch

- warm joints

- get body and brain ready for more intense exercises

**The Body Of The Class
"LET'S ENERGIZE" and
"LET'S TONE UP"**

The body of the class is the "meat and potatoes" of the fitness class. It is during this segment that the most intense effort is required from the participants.

During the body of the class, you will work on different elements of fitness such as aerobic exercises (walking, climbing stairs, etc.) and strength (sit ups, arm pulls, etc.).

What can you do to improve the fitness level of your participants?

**The Aerobic Portion
"LET'S ENERGIZE"**

In this part of the class, you should use the large muscle groups of the body in moderate to strenuous exercise.

Interval Training

One method used to develop the aerobic aspect of fitness is interval training. Interval training is repetitive aerobic exercise where participants perform endurance tasks (e.g. a dance) for a short period of time. This activity is immediately followed by a period in which participants will be able to recover while doing a light activity such as walking slowly. Following the resting period, participants will continue with a dance or a game. Interval training is a very effective method to improve the cardiovascular system. Taking the time to rest between two peaks of activity lessens the chance of injury as the participants do not tire as easily.

The Games

When introducing a game to the participants it is important to keep the rules simple. Remember that the purpose of games in a fitness class is to help participants develop their aerobic capacity along with other elements of fitness (range of motion and strength) in a pleasant and informal setting. A game should be structured in such a way that every participant has a chance to play and enjoy themselves. For example, introducing beach balls in a volleyball game could add an element of fun. In Section 3 several games are introduced that work well in a seniors' fitness class.

Dance is another activity that should be included in your fitness programme. Through dance it is possible to work on the aerobic component along with other elements of fitness (range of motion, aerobic fitness, strength). The choice of music is very important when planning a dance activity. Participants follow the rhythm and speed of the music when dancing. It is important to remember that the faster the music, the harder the activity. When choosing music, keep in mind the fitness level of your participants.

For The Strength Portion "LET'S TONE UP"

The development of strength is very important and should be part of any fitness programme. When developing strength, the emphasis is placed on muscle toning. Strength exercises will help your muscles become more efficient and less vulnerable to accidents and injuries. Please remember that strength exercises should be introduced with caution since participants have a tendency to hold their breath during these exercises. Participants should be reminded to breathe normally during exercise. Strength exercises can be done using either the participant's own body weight or by using light weights such as sand bottles or the weights introduced in Chapter 6.

Remember:
The body of the class should be a mixture of new and old activities. The introduction of new activities should be at a slow pace to make sure that the exercise is understood and performed well by all participants.

The Cool-Down Period "LET'S STRETCH" and "LET'S RELAX"

The cool-down period has two main purposes:

- to gradually allow the body to get rid of excess heat

- to work on greater flexibility

The cool-down period should last 10 minutes or more following the more intense exercises during the body of the class.

Continuing light exercise such as walking will help the body to slowly return to a normal internal temperature.

Stretching exercises (**"LET'S STRETCH"**) help recovery and counter soreness and tightness possibly caused by intense activities. In a cool-down period, stretching exercises should be more intense than during the warm-up period because the body is completely warmed up and ready to stretch more than when the muscles are cooler.

A cool-down period should include:

- a gradual decrease or tapering off of the aerobic intensity

- a mixture of reduced aerobic activity and stretching activities (walking slowly, ankle stretches, etc.)

A cool-down period should be related to the intensity of the body of the class. The harder the body of the class, the longer the cool-down.

The Relaxation Period "LET'S RELAX"

The relaxation period is the last part of the cool-down period. These activities are aimed at helping participants reach their resting heart rate while relaxing muscles, tendons and ligaments that have worked progressively harder since the beginning of the warm-up period. The relaxation period should last between 10 and 15 minutes.

During the relaxation period you should:

- help the participants to find a comfortable position, e.g. lying down on their back in a quiet area; this activity should be done on a towel or mat as the floor may be dusty or cool

- encourage participants to close their eyes

- allow participants to become aware of their resting state while encouraging deep breathing

- turn down the lights to ensure a better resting atmosphere

- help the participants to immobilize and relax each part of their body, starting from the feet and moving up to the head

- help the participants allow their ideas to flow freely through their mind; be careful when suggesting any particular type of idea such as "imagine you are on a beach…"; this practice may stress beginners when trying to relax; the most important element for beginners is to get acquainted with the feeling of being relaxed

The Closure Of The Class

The closure of the class is equally as important as the introduction of the class. During the last few minutes of class, the instructor should take the time to encourage and praise the participants. Feedback from the participants can also be gathered and is essential in order to adapt your activities to their individual needs and expectations.

This last period of class is also important since it provides the instructor and the participants with a chance to socialize and to discuss in amore relaxed manner. Through these informal discussions, you, as an instructor, can get to know your participants better.

Preparing Class Material

Prior to teaching a class it is important to plan and prepare the material that will be needed. A list of materials should be written down before entering the class.

Arrive early to class so you have time to prepare the materials and to welcome your participants.

Participants should take part in the organization of materials for the class as much as possible. This practice will maximize the organization time, while keeping everyone involved.

During class, if a participant is out of breath, ask him to get some material or equipment for you. This will force him/her to slow down.

Music is an important part of a fitness class. Proper music can motivate participants to be more active, while adding to the atmosphere of the class.

Music should be chosen with care; participants will tend to adjust the rhythm of their movements to the music. Music with a rhythm that is too fast could be dangerous for beginners.

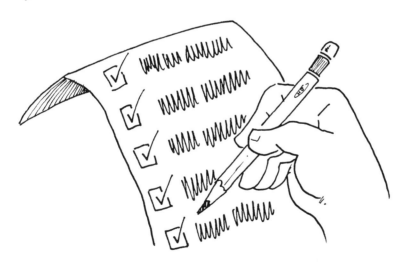

Music should be chosen according to the type of activity (game, relaxation, etc.) and the level of the participants.

Music should be changed on a regular basis. It is important to vary the type of music in order to keep a note of novelty in the class. You should have a variety of musical tapes for different levels of participants and for different types of activities — the warm-up, games, relaxation, etc.

TEACHING THE CLASS

Now that you have prepared the material and equipment needed for your class, you are ready to start teaching. The aim, at this stage, is to ensure that the participants will feel interested and rewarded by the activities. Some things to keep in mind while teaching a class are:

- keep constant communication between participants and the instructors at all times

- be aware of the behaviour of participants

- be sure to modify and adapt material and exercises according to the situation

The Art of Communicating

Verbal Communication

The choice of words is basic to good communication during the class. The instructor should choose terms that are natural and easily understood by the participants. Complicated words do not necessarily mean a better class — it is better to use simple expressions and words.

As participants age, some sounds are harder to hear. Instructors using a high-pitched voice are more difficult to understand. Be near participants when you speak. Speak loudly enough for them to hear and don't speak too quickly.

When giving explanations to the participants, turn down the music and try to avoid background noises as much as possible. Some participants may find it difficult to concentrate on verbal information while listening to background noise.

Before giving instructions, make sure you have the attention of all the participants. To get their attention you may try:

- clapping your hands

- turning the lights on and off

- using a whistle

- turning the music on or off

- standing quietly until all participants are watching you

Non-Verbal Communication

Gestures, facial expressions and demonstrations, are all non-verbal ways that support or, in many cases, replace the spoken word. Gestures such as touching, smiling, laughing, will add warmth to the atmosphere of the class.

Each verbal explanation should be supported by non-verbal elements when possible.

Demonstrations should be done slowly and as carefully as possible especially when demonstrating and explaining a new exercise.

The Art Of Observing The Class

The first and foremost important observation to be made by the instructor during a class is to watch for warning signs. Signs of tiredness and exertion have to be identified quickly and action must be taken immediately.

Watching the participants' behaviour and reactions during class will give an indication of how well participants are becoming involved. One objective of a fitness class should be to get participants involved as much as possible in the different activities offered. If participants are involved in the activities and exercises presented during the class, it is an indication of a high level of interest on their part.

How To Do Quick Adaptations During Teaching

In many cases, participants do not respond to an activity or an exercise the way the instructor anticipated. Therefore quick adaptations and changes have to be made on the spot. In order to make those changes, here are some guidelines.

Changing the activity or exercise

Activities or exercises are tools to help the instructor achieve the objectives of the class. You should not be afraid to modify or change an exercise if the participants do not seem comfortable with it. A good plan is to have a few back-up activities or exercises in case the ones chosen do not have the expected impact on the participants. Always be flexible in your teaching!

Changing the pace of the exercise

An exercise or activity is often not well accepted because it is either too easy or too difficult for the participants. By speeding up or slowing down a game, dance, or an exercise, you could make a big difference in the response from the participants to this activity.

Varying material

A change of material during exercises, games or dances, could have a positive effect on the activity and make your class more enjoyable. Do not be afraid to introduce novel ideas, different kinds of balls or a new music rhythm to a game or exercise.

Teaching Tricks

The art of teaching or helping participants learn or improve new movement, exercises, games or dances is a personal experience in which the instructor will adapt his/her teaching to his/her strengths. Since we all have strengths and weaknesses the following 'tricks' could help enhance your teaching.

Team Teaching

Team teaching is an excellent method of maximizing the teaching impact. Team teaching is a situation where two or more instructors share the teaching of a class. This practice helps capitalize on the instructors' strengths and abilities. Different ways of structuring team teaching are:

- to have each instructor introduce activities to the group alternately

- to have each instructor take charge of different sections of the class (the introduction, the warm-up, the body of the class, the cool-down, the closure)

Teaching Notes

When preparing your class, it is important to make some notes of what you want to teach and accomplish during a particular class. Teaching notes should be written on cards or sheets that could be easily carried during class. Some instructors like to carry their notes on a string around their neck. These notes could include:

- exercises to be taught and their order of presentation

- important notes such as upcoming events and personal notes on participants, e.g. birthdays, anniversaries

- important notes for the instructor, e.g. different warning signs, emergency telephone numbers, organizational notes

Partner Work (Buddy System)
With this practice, participants are always working in pairs. Encouraging participants to work in pairs (except when stretching) is not only a way to help them maintain their level of motivation during class, but it is also a safety procedure. By working in pairs, participants can keep an eye on each other for warning signs.

Body Checks

Talking and Singing
This is used to ensure that the activities of the class are not too intense for the participants. To conduct this body check, stand beside the participants and talk to them. If the participants are able to carry on a conversation or sing a few notes, they have passed the check. If they are so breathless that they can only use one-syllable words, then you should decrease the intensity of the activity for those individuals. Slow down the activity or change the exercise if necessary. This same check could be performed between participants, therefore conversation should be encouraged during exercise periods. If you exercise alone, the same body check could be used except that you would sing out loud.

This body check is very convenient; you do not have to stop the class and it will provide you with some information on how the class is able to cope with the level of intensity of the exercises.

The Target Heart Rate

The target heart rate is another important body check. On a regular basis participants should verify their heart rate (please consult Chapter 6 for more information on the appropriate procedure to follow).

The result of this check should be matched with the suggested target heart rate for the participant. If the heart rate is higher than suggested, then the intensity of the activity should be decreased.

While Moving During Class

As an instructor, walk in the opposite direction of the participants.

Be sure that participants can see you at all times.

Do not stand in the participant's peripheral field of vision.

Maximizing Exercise Space

When planning fitness activities, it is important to maximize the space available to you during the class. This practice will add spice to the activities and help break the monotony of routine exercises. Some activities might be better performed with the group in a circle, (e.g. stretching exercises), having groups of three participants working in a triangle (e.g. passing a ball to each other), or following different pathways (e.g. a game situation). Examples of different space set-ups that could be used during a class are presented in FIGURE 2.

Interaction Between Participants and Instructors

Interaction between participants and instructors refers to the relationship between teacher and participant during the class. Mutual respect between instructors and participants tends to foster better results and a more enjoyable atmosphere.

Instructors should always be open to participants' suggestions and reactions. Input from them could be important to improving the quality of the class.

The participants should be encouraged to participate at their own pace.

The importance of feedback is often overlooked during a class. A feedback is how the instructor reacts to an action (exercise, movement, etc.) from the participant. Feedback should be given immediately after the exercise and should be specific rather than general.

FIGURE 2

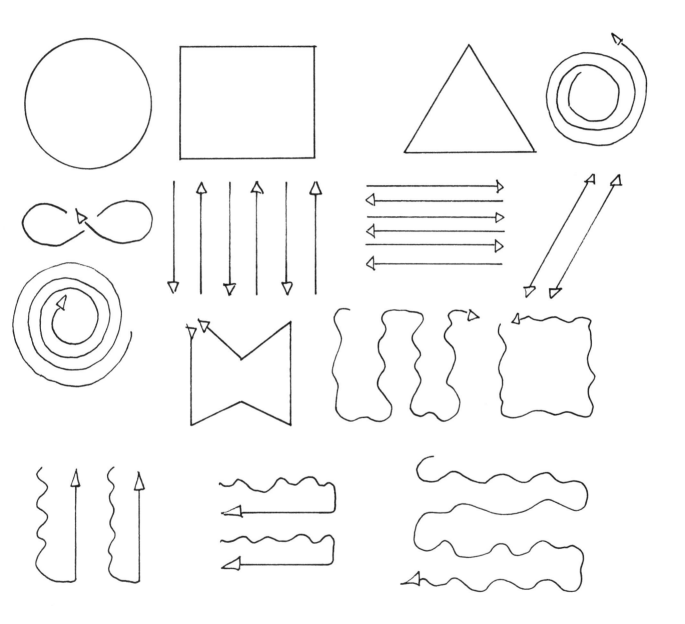

Specific feedback would be:
"Try to lift your leg a bit higher in this exercise."

General feedback would be:
"You performed the exercise very well."

Specific feedback tends to be more helpful to the participants than general feedback since it gives the participants specific instructions on how they can improve.

After Class Evaluation

What Is Class Evaluation?

Class evaluation is made following a teaching session. This activity is designed to see if the objectives planned for the class were met. Looking back at the class, the instructor may ask himself the following questions:

Have I met the objectives I set for that class?

Were the activities appropriate for the level of the participants?

How could the achievement of the participants be measured?

Was the teaching method used during class appropriate for the level and expectations of the participants?

Was the reaction of the participants positive? What kind of feedback did I receive during or after class?

In order to answer these questions, the instructor could use different evaluation methods. Among the possible evaluation methods are:

Feedback from Participants

This approach consists of asking the participants, either through questionnaires or discussion, how they would grade the class. Information from the participants regarding the class can also be gathered by means of observation. You will be able to see how participants enjoyed the activity.

Perception of the Instructor

This approach consists of having you, the instructor, make note of your impressions following the class. One method of keeping track of your observations is by building a log-book. The log-book is a personal notebook that helps you look back and evaluate past classes. Notes relating to the exercises and activities as well as reactions of the participants toward activities could be recorded in this book.

Changes To Be Made To The Class Preparation

Following the evaluation period the instructor can establish what changes should be made for future classes. These changes are made to improve

the teaching of the programme and to fulfill the objectives of the class.

Teaching a fitness class is a challenging and rewarding experience. Careful preparation of your teaching material and equipment is needed in order to maximize your efforts. Remember that

the participants should always be the centre of attention in a fitness class. It is therefore essential to observe their reactions to the activities in order to adapt your programme accordingly.

CONCLUSION

The previous sections addressed planning and teaching a fitness programme. All of the elements discussed were carefully chosen to help you, as an instructor, plan and teach a fitness session for seniors. You should always be open to the participants' reactions and invlovement within the programme since this precious feedback will help you readjust your programme to their needs and expectations.

References

Berridge, M. E., & Wand G. R. (1987). International perspectives on adapted physical activity. Champagne, Ill. Human Kinetics Publishers Inc.

Brunelle, J., Drouin, D., Godbout, P., Morin, G., & Tousignant, M. (ed.). (1988). La supervision de l'intervention en activité physique. Montréal, QC.

Corbin, C. B., Dowell, L. J., Lindsey H. (1978). Tolson concepts in physical education: With laboratories and experiments (3rd ed.). Dubuque, Iowa: Win C. Brown Company Publisher.

DiGennaro, J. (1983). The new physical fitness: Exercise for everybody. Englewood, Colorado: Morton Publishing Company.

Kraus, R. G. (1985). Recreation program planning today. Glenview, Ill: Scott, Foresman and Company.

Lundegren, H. M., Farrell, P. (1985). Evaluation for leisure service managers: A dynamic approach. Montreal: Saunders College Publishing.

Shevers, J. S., Faib, H. F. (1980). Recreational service for the aging. Philadelphia: Lea & Febeger.

Teaff, J. D. (1985). Leisure services with the elderly. Toronto: Mosby College Publishing.

Section 3

GAMES

We cannot underestimate the added dimension that playing games brings to each exercise class. They have the benefit of increasing our heart rate and working our heart and lungs, but more than that they bring enjoyment, laughter and social interaction that are so important to the older adult. Games should be introduced during the "LET'S ENERGIZE" portion of the exercise class and should be promoted as cooperative, not competitive. By introducing games to your class, you will see and enjoy a new side of your participants.

The following section suggests some games to play with your participants. Join in and have fun!

Game #1
UP WITH BALLOONS:

Each participant is given a balloon. The object of this exercise is to keep the balloon up in the air. To make this more difficult, the participants may use just their heads, feet or elbows, etc., instead of their hands.

This game can also be played with partners.

Game #2
INNER LEG SQUEEZE:

Mark two parallel lines on the floor with tape, approximately 10 feet (3m) apart. Divide participants into teams with approximately six players in each.

Have the leader of each team line up on one of the marked lines with other team members behind.

The leader of each team is given a sponge. The sponge is to be placed in between the thighs, just above the knees. While squeezing the sponge with inner thigh muscles and with no help from hands, players must walk to the opposite line and back without dropping the sponge. If the sponge is dropped, return to starting position and do it again. If successfully completed, pass the sponge to the next person on the team.

When all members of the team have had a turn with the sponge, do the same with a ball and then with balloons.

Game #3
SPACE ORIENTATION:

Form a large circle. Have every second person take two steps forward into the circle, forming a circle within a circle.

Pick one person to start weaving in and out around the participants. The person next to the leader starts to weave when the leader is two people from the starting position.

All participants follow in the same manner until you have continuous movement.

Game #4
OBSTACLE COURSE:

Divide the group into teams. Set up an obstacle course using tables, chairs, boxes, ropes, etc. The participants must go around, under and through them without touching the obstacles.

When the course is completed by one participant, the next member of the team starts the course, and so on.

Game #5
CIRCLE KICK:

Form a circle.

The object is to pass the ball around the circle using a soccer-type kick. Try to keep the ball inside the circle.

More balls may be added.

Game #6
MUSICAL HOOPS:

This game is the same as the traditional musical chairs but the participants must stand inside a hoop.

Game #7
BEANBAG RACE:

Place two lines of tape on the floor approximately 10 feet (3m) apart.

Divide participants into teams. Team members line up behind their leader. The leader places a beanbag (sponge) on top of his head, walks to the opposite line and returns to place the beanbag (sponge) on the next team member's head.

Repeat until all team members have had a turn.

Game #8
ODD SHOES:

All participants sit in a circle and remove their shoes. The instructor picks up shoes and scatters them all around the room. On a signal, participants must find their shoes, put them on, and sit back down in the circle.

Game #9
NAME GAME:

Place one person in the centre of a circle with a ball. The person in the centre calls out a name and passes the ball to that person. These two people must then exchange places. Repeat.

To increase the action and fun, add more balls and people in the middle. Passes in the air or bounce passes are fine.

Game #10
CLOTHESPINS AND COLOURS:

This game is played very similarly to the game of musical chairs.

The instructor attaches clothespins to the back of chairs, to the curtains, etc. (these chairs with the clothespins are placed in the centre of the circle, evenly spaced). The participants are instructed to form a circle and to walk counter-clockwise in that circle to the music. The instructor calls out a colour and stops the music. The participants must then find someone who is wearing that colour, get a clothespin and attach it to that person's article of clothing in that colour.

Continue the game until all the clothespins are used. The winner? Person with the most clothespins!

Game #11
BEACH BALL BOOGIE:

Have all participants find a partner. Half of the class is given balls and is instructed to place the balls between themselves and their partner — stomach to stomach, side to side, head to head, behind to behind, forehead to chest, and so on. Do not hold onto the balls with your hands!

When the music begins, all the partners with beach balls dance to the beat. When the instructor says, 'change', participants pass their beach balls (without using their hands) to their nearest partner. Those not connected by a beach ball dance to the beat while waiting to receive a ball.

More interesting: change partners with the balls or boogie in fours with two balls.

Game #12
PING PONG PASS :
(A good game for arthritic hands)

Players are lined up in two or more equal teams for this amusing relay race. Five ping pong balls are placed in a container that is placed at the end of each line — an empty container is placed at the other end. Players clasp hands with the person on either side. Hands must remain clasped throughout the game.

The first player of each team picks up the ball with their free hand and passes it to his other hand, which is clasped with the hand of the second player. The ball is passed down the entire line and the last player puts the ball in the container with his free hand.

As soon as the first player has passed the first ball, he picks up another and continues to pick up and pass all five balls as quickly as possible. If a ball is dropped, it must be picked up by the pair of players who dropped it without unclasping their hands. The team to get all of the balls in the container at the foot of the line wins.

Game #13
BOMBING THE BALL:

Form two teams with the same number of participants on each team.

Have the teams facing each other in the formation shown below.

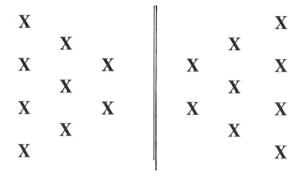

Place a beach ball on a line drawn between the two teams. Give each participant a bean bag.

On a signal, the participants 'bomb' the beach ball, trying to make the ball end up in the opposing team's territory. Each participant only gets to throw their bean bag once. If the ball ends up on the opposing player's side, the team scores a point.

Game #14

FOX AND SQUIRREL:

Players stand in a circle facing inward.

Two tennis balls represent two squirrels.

One bean bag represents a fox.

The fox tries to catch the squirrels.

In order to do this, players pass the balls to the player beside them, always continuing in the same direction.

The fox is thrown <u>across</u> the circle from one player to the next. The fox tries to catch up with the squirrel. The goal of the game is to avoid one person having the fox and the squirrel at one time.

The instructor, to make it more interesting, can call out 'change directions.'

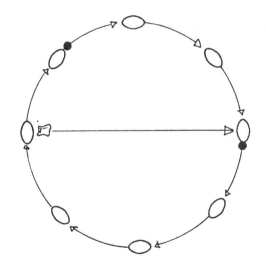

Squirrels go around the circle
Fox is thrown 'across' the circle

SIMPLE EQUIPMENT

EQUIPMENT	USE
Nylons, Pantihose	Place one end of nylon in one hand, the the other end in your other hand, S T R E T C H. Place hands behind back, hold nylon in each hand, lift arms up. Stand on one end of pantihose; with your hands, pull on the other end. Make knots in nylons.
Uncooked Spaghetti	Pick up one piece at a time and put it in a container with a small opening.
Marbles	Pick up marbles with toes and put into a container. Roll marbles between the palms of your hands.
Clothespins	Squeeze the clothespins between your thumb and 1. forefinger 2. middle finger 3. ring finger 4. baby finger Repeat with the other hand.
Metal Clothes Hanger	Form clothes hanger into a circle and cover it with a nylon sock. This makes a great badminton racket!
Bean Bags/Bag of Peas	Balance bean bags on your head while you walk. Use to throw at a target or into a container.

SIMPLE EQUIPMENT

EQUIPMENT	USE
Bicycle Inner Tube	Place inner tube in hands and then take off the valve S T R E T C H and tie with a knot. Place inner tube under your feet, hold onto the ends with your hands and S T R E T C H. Attach to a door knob or the leg of a dresser or bed and S T R E T C H.

GLOSSARY OF TERMS

Keeping with the goal of this manual, medical and confusing terms have been kept to a minimum whenever possible. Wherever the use of these words is necessary or cannot be avoided, they have been included in this list to avoid confusion.

The explanation of the terms in this glossary are in no way meant to be complete dictionary definitions, but merely an aid to help the reader understand these terms in the context that they are used.

Acid
A substance which helps break down food for digestion.

Aneurysm
A weak spot on the artery wall which fills with blood and balloons outward (like an inflated inner tube with a weak spot).

Angina
Recurring chest pain brought on by physical or emotional stress.

Aphasia
An impairment of the body's ability to communicate through speech, writing or signs. Aphasia is often caused by stroke.

Arteriosclerosis
A disease which causes the artery walls to thicken and lose their elasticity. This may cause other heart problems such as heart attack or high blood pressure.

Artery
Elastic tube-like structure which transports blood to the lungs and other parts of the body.

Arthritis
A general term used for problems of the body's joints and surrounding tissues.

Atherosclerosis
A buildup of fatty deposits (e.g., cholesterol) in the arteries. This may cause other problems such as high blood pressure or heart attack.

Autoimmune Disease
A disease in which your body is attacked by its own defence system (immune system).

Bacteria
Microscopic (too small to see), simple single cell structure that can cause infections or disease.

Bacterial Infection
A term used to describe the result of harmful bacteria entering the body.

Ballistic Exercise/Movement
An exercise/movement in which there is a quick or sharp motion.

Basic Position
Stand up straight, look straight ahead, feet shoulder-width apart, knees slightly bent, and arms hanging loosely alongside body (see chapter 6).

Blood Circulation
See Blood Flow

Blood Clot
Thickening of the blood into a solid matter which impairs blood flow within the blood vessel.

Blood Flow
The flow of blood through the blood vessels.

Blood Pressure
The pressure exerted on the walls of the blood vessels by the blood (see chapter 2, section 3).

Blood Vessels
Small tubes which carry blood throughout the body.

Bone Mass
The amount of bone in the body.

Bone Density
A term which usually refers to the weight and strength of bone.

Calcium
A substance which is important for healthy bones and teeth. Milk is a good source of calcium.

Carbon Dioxide
A substance which your cells produce when they use up oxygen. Carbon dioxide is part of the air that you breathe out.

Cardiopulmonary Resuscitation
An emergency first aid technique used for heart attack victims who have stopped breathing and whose heart has stopped. "CPR" is designed to get the victim breathing and the heart pumping.

Cardiovascular Disease
Illness which affects the heart and blood vessels (see chapter 2, section 3).

Cartilage
A tough material which cushions and protects the ends of bones. (e.g., the shiny white part on the end of a chicken leg).

Cell
The smallest living unit of the human body. Your body is made up of cells.

Cholesterol
A fatty substance which sticks to the inner walls of arteries and may cause cardiovascular disease.

Chronic
Recurring, continuous or persistent (e.g. arthritis is a chronic disease).

Congestive Heart Failure
A condition in which the heart becomes weak and unable to pump enough blood to meet the needs of the body.

Cornea
A clear outer layer of the eye which helps in focusing.

Deformed
Misshapen or unusually out of proper shape.

Degenerating
Decay or worsening of condition.

Degenerative
A condition that causes a worsening of physical or mental qualities.

Deteriorating
See Degenerating.

Diabetes
A condition which causes the body to not use or control the amount of sugar (glucose) in the blood. There are two types of diabetes - Type I and Type II.

Diaphragm
A thin, flat muscle which separates the chest from the abdomen and helps in breathing.

Disease
A sickness of the body or mind.

Disorder
A condition in which a part (or parts) of the body does not function normally or properly.

Ear Canal
The section of the ear which runs from the outside to the inner ear.

Efficiency
The production of the desired effects or results with minimum waste of time, effort or skill.

Elasticity
The ability to stretch and return to its original shape. Usually refers to muscles or other tissues.

Endurance
The ability to withstand prolonged exercise.

Enzymes
Substances which help break down food for digestion.

Excretion
The removal of wastes from the body.

Exercise Class
In the exercise section of this manual, an exercise class refers to one exercise workout, whether it be as a group exercising with a fitness instructor or a person exercising alone.

Exercising Pulse Rate
The speed at which your heart beats while you are exercising. (seeTraining Heart Rate Zone Chart in chapter 6).

Fatigue
Weariness which may be brought on by physical exertion, depression, sickness or other factors.

Field of Vision
The area that you can see without moving your eyes.

Flexibility

The range of motion through which a joint or group of joints are able to move.

Fracture
Break or crack of a bone.

Gangrene
The decay of body tissue due to an obstruction in the blood flow such as a blood clot.

Genetic
Caused by heredity.

Glucose
A type of sugar which occurs naturally in foods such as fruits and honey. It is a source of energy for the body.

Hair Follicles
Small sac - shaped secretory gland or cavity containing hair root.

Heart Rate
The rate at which the heart beats; measured in beats per minute.

Heart Attack
A condition in which the blood flow to a part of the heart is blocked. This results in the death of that part of the heart.

Hormone
A substance which the body produces to control some functions in the body.

Hormone Deficiency
A lacking of a certain hormone.

Hyperventilation
An increased amount of air entering the lungs resulting in excess loss of carbon dioxide from the body. Can cause dizziness and/or fainting.

Immune System
The body's defence system which fights off bacteria and diseases.

Indigestion
A problem with the digestion of food. This often causes stomach upset.

Inflammation
Swelling, redness, heat and pain in a certain area of the body caused by infections or diseases.

Insulin
A hormone which controls the sugar level in the blood.

Intestine
A long, winding tube which goes from the stomach to the rectum and helps in the digestion and absorption of food. The length of the intestines is about 26 feet (8 metres).

Isometric Exercises
Exercises in which there is no change in the length of the muscle or muscles involved (no movement of this part of the body) i.e., pushing against a wall.

Joint
A meeting of two bones which allows for movement of different parts of the body.

Juvenile Diabetes(Type I diabetes).
A type of diabetes in which the body does not produce insulin.

Labia
Lips of female genitals.

Ligament
A band of tissue which holds bones and organs in place and holds joints together (see diagram chapter 2, section 1).

Locked Knees
Legs fully extended (straight).

Lubricating Fluid
A substance which oils joints to make movement smoother.

Maturity-onset Diabetes (Type II diabetes).
A type of diabetes in which the body does not properly use insulin. This type of diabetes is often attributed to the aging process.

Metabolic Rate
The speed at which nutritious food is chemically changed into living matter.

Metabolism
Process, in organism or single cell, by which nutritious material is built up into living matter.

Mucous
A slimy substance secreted by the body such as saliva.

Muscle Group
A group of muscles which work together to make a specific movement, e.g. bending your leg.

Muscles
Elastic tissues that work together to move the bones by contracting and relaxing.

Nerves
Small tissue conductors which carry messages between the brain and parts of the body.

Nutrients
Food used by the cells to produce energy.

Organ
A group of tissues which work together to perform a specific function, e.g. liver.

Osteoarthritis
A condition affecting the joints in which there is a degeneration of cartilage.

Osteoporosis
A condition in which there is a gradual bone loss, causing the bones to become brittle and easily broken.

Oxygen
A component of air which is used by the cells to produce energy. Oxygen is part of the air that we breathe in.

Pancreas
An organ located near the stomach which produces digestive juices and insulin.

Particles
Objects which are too small to see with the naked eye, e.g. dust

Periodontal
Tissues surrounding the teeth (gums).

Peripheral Vision
What can be seen on the edges of the field of vision. i.e. the edges or fringe of your vision.

Pigment
Natural colouring - matter of animal or plant tissue, e.g. pigment produces brown or white skin.

Pinched Nerve
Compression of the root or fibre of the nerve.

Pores
Small openings in the skin through which fluids such as sweat may pass.

Post-Menopausal
Referring to a woman who has passed menopause.

Prolonged Strength Exercises
An exercise in which there is a continued contraction of the muscles.

Pulse Rate
The rate at which your heart beats; measured in beats per minute.

Pupil
The black spot in the centre of the eye which regulates the passage of light.

Range of Motion
The degree that a joint may rotate or move.

Recovery Pulse Rate
The elevated rate at which your heart beats after exercising.

Rectum
The lowest segment of the large intestine (see chapter 1, section 6).

Remission
A period in which no symptoms of a chronic disease are apparent.

Repetitions
The number of times an exercise is repeated.

Resting Pulse Rate
see Resting Heart Rate

Resting Heart Rate
The rate at which your heart beats while the body is at rest.

Rheumatoid Arthritis
A condition which affects many of the body's systems. There are many symptoms including pain and swelling in the joints, weakness and possible joint deformity.

Session
In the exercise section of this manual, a session refers to a complete exercise workout performed 3 times per week for 4 weeks.

Skeletal Mass
The amount of bone in the body.

Skin Pigment
A substance which gives skin its colour and protects it from the sun.

Spinal Cord
A part of the central nervous system which is housed by the backbone.

Stimulants
Agents that arouse organic activity, strengthen the action of the heart, increase vitality and promote a sense of well-being.

Stroke
A condition in which there is lack of blood going to a certain part of the brain. This causes the possible death of that part of the brain.

Sweat Glands
Very small organs located beneath the skin which produce sweat.

Talk Test
A simple test which tells you if you are exercising too hard. If you are unable to keep up a conversation, or can only speak in one-syllable words, you are exercising too hard.

Target Heart Rate
A heart rate zone (determined by age) which helps determine a safe level for exercising (see the Target Heart Rate Zone Chart in chapter 6).

Tendon
Tough strong tissue which attaches muscle to bone.

Tissue
Cells of the same type which work together to perform a function.

Ulcer
An open sore often found inside the digestive system, e.g. stomach ulcer.

Vaginal
Belonging to the genital canal in the female, extending from the uterus to the vulva.

Valsalva Maneuver
Holding the breath during exercise. This causes an increased pressure in the chest, resulting in poorer efficiency of the heart. This may cause serious problems such as heart attacks or strokes.

Varicose Veins
A condition in which the veins are
visibly enlarged or swollen.

Vein
Thin tube-like structure which
transports blood to the heart from the
lungs and other parts of
the body.

Vertebrae
The segments of the backbone.

Vertebral Column
The backbone.

Virus
A microscopic (too small to see) germ
which can cause infection or disease.

Windpipe
The tube that goes from the mouth to
the lungs.

CONTRIBUTORS

This book was made possible through the collaborative effort of the following people:

Manual Committee Members

Staff:
Yvonne Wagorn, Coordinator, Positive Health for Seniors

Sonia Théberge, Project Officer, Positive Health for Seniors

Volunteers:
Chairperson - William A.R. Orban, B.Sc., M.S., Ph.D., LL.D., F.A.C.S.M., Exercise Physiologist

Dianne Parker-Taillon, B.Sc.P.T., M.Sc. (Kin.)

Dale Edwards, B.Sc.P.T., R.P.T.

Sharon Hudson, R.N.

Jennifer Godfrey, B.P.E., M.P.E. (Admin.)

Rolland Champagne, fitness instructor, Positive Health for Seniors

Thérèse Larocque, fitness instructor, Positive Health for Seniors

Aubert Séguin, participant, Positive Health for Seniors

Henri Groulx, participant, Positive Health for Seniors

Jean Hurtubise, participant, Positive Health for Seniors

Researcher and Writers:
Doug Scullion, B.Sc. Major in Biochemistry, B.Sc. Major in Exercise Science, candidate M.Sc.

François Gravelle, M.E.P. (Admin.), Graduate Student Ph.D., Major in Physical Activity (pedagogy) for Seniors

Gilles Hébert, B.A., Candidate Ph.D. Psy.

J.C. Pageot, Ph.D., Chairman, Department of Leisure Studies, University of Ottawa; Chairman, National Advisory Council, Secretariat for Fitness in the Third Age

Christine Dalgity, student, St. Lawrence College

Paul Wagorn, student, University of Waterloo

Pamela Willis, student, University of Victoria

<u>**Reviewers and Contributors**</u>

Reviewers:
The Arthritis Society, Ottawa

Yvan Lavoie, M.D.

C. Doug Smith, M.D., F.R.C.P.(C)

Sylvie Théberge, M.Ps.

Pauline Witherly-Manuel, Public Relations, OSTOP Ottawa, Osteoporosis Support Group

Contributors:
Janet Chambers, Manager, Senior Services, Canadian Red Cross Society

Diane Cloutier, student of Kinanthropology, University of Ottawa

Danielle Dagenais, Executive Secretary, Élisabeth Bruyère Health Centre

Zelda Freedman, B.A., librarian, Élisabeth Bruyère Health Centre

Donna Lordon, B.Nsg., D.P.H.N., B.A.(Pol. Sc. and Eng.), M.H.A., C.H.E.

Janice Miller, B.Sc., P.T., Assistant Director, Physiotherapy, Heart Institute Prevention and Rehabilitation Centre, Ottawa Civic Hospital, Ottawa

Paul Parent, Assistant Executive Director/Communications, Élisabeth Bruyère Health Centre

France Pérodeau, D.C., Clinque Chiropratique de Hull

Frank Reardon, B.Sc., M.Sc., Ph.D., Associate Professor, Human Kinetics, Faculty of Health Sciences, University of Ottawa

Louise Tetrault, B.A., B.Sc.Hon., M.D., C.C.F.P.

Carole Villeneuve, R.P.Dt., Manager, Clinical Nutrition Service, Élisabeth Bruyère Health Centre

Guidance was provided by:

Advisory Committee, Positive Health for Seniors

Chairperson: Richard Reardon, retired Chief Telecommunications and Electronics Policy and Regulations, Canadian Coast Guard

Dr. Denise Allard, Chair, Educational Policies, Faculty of Health Sciences, University of Ottawa and Gerontologist

Gabriel Blouin, Associate Broker, Real Estate, semi-retired

Dr. Wilma Dare, Trustee, Élisabeth Bruyère Health Centre

Rita Lemick, Programme Officer, Health Promotion Directorate, Health and Welfare, Canada

Donna Lordon, Assistant Executive Director of Clinical Services, Élisabeth Bruyère Health Centre

Dr. William Orban, retired Professor of Kinanthropology

Norma Strachan, Project Manager, Medication Awareness Project, Council on Aging, Ottawa-Carleton

Jean-Paul Van Bergen, fitness instructor, Positive Health for Seniors, St. Bernardin

Dr. Beatrice Wickett, Psychologist, Palliative Care Unit, Élisabeth Bruyère Health Centre